# Islam, Development, and Urban Women's Reproductive Practices

Drawing on fieldwork conducted in Rabat, Morocco, this ethnography analyzes the relationship between neoliberal development policies, urban women's reproductive practices, and popular understandings of Islam. In the 1990s, Morocco shifted its attention from economic to human development, as economic reforms in the preceding decades ultimately did not address social issues such as access to healthcare and education and poverty. Development programs like the National Initiative for Human Development seek to create modern citizens who are responsible, self-sustaining, and will make choices that better their well-being. Hughes Rinker considers the implications that the reorientation from primarily economic to social development has on reproductive healthcare. Drawing on observations in health clinics; interviews with patients, medical staff, and at government and development agencies; and a document analysis, she demonstrates how women appropriate the medical practices and spaces of intervention aimed at creating modern citizens to form new religious identities, novel ideas of motherhood, and interpretations of neoliberal citizenship based on Islamic beliefs. Women's interpretations of Islam are not incompatible with the state's agenda for modernization, but rather serve as rationale for women to accept modern reproductive practices, such as contraception, ultrasounds, and pregnancy tests. However, even though female patients appropriate medical practices, they reinscribe development tropes that suggest they participate in modernization through their reproductive bodies and mothering instead of their productive labor. Hughes Rinker complicates neoliberalism as she shows it is unproductive to have a set conceptualization of neoliberal citizens, and more productive to examine the practices and discourses that create such citizens.

**Cortney Hughes Rinker** earned her Ph.D. in Sociocultural Anthropology from the University of California Irvine. She is Assistant Professor in the Department of Sociology and Anthropology at George Mason University.

## Routledge Studies in Anthropology

1 **Student Mobility and Narrative in Europe**
The New Strangers
*Elizabeth Murphy-Lejeune*

2 **The Question of the Gift**
Essays across Disciplines
*Edited by Mark Osteen*

3 **Decolonising Indigenous Rights**
*Edited by Adolfo de Oliveira*

4 **Traveling Spirits**
Migrants, Markets and Mobilities
*Edited by Gertrud Hüwelmeier and Kristine Krause*

5 **Anthropologists, Indigenous Scholars and the Research Endeavour**
Seeking Bridges Towards Mutual Respect
*Edited by Joy Hendry and Laara Fitznor*

6 **Confronting Capital**
Critique and Engagement in Anthropology
*Edited by Pauline Gardiner Barber, Belinda Leach and Winnie Lem*

7 **Adolescent Identity**
Evolutionary, Cultural and Developmental Perspectives
*Edited by Bonnie L. Hewlett*

8 **The Social Life of Climate Change Models**
Anticipating Nature
*Edited by Kirsten Hastrup and Martin Skrydstrup*

9 **Islam, Development, and Urban Women's Reproductive Practices**
*Cortney Hughes Rinker*

# Islam, Development, and Urban Women's Reproductive Practices

Cortney Hughes Rinker

Routledge
Taylor & Francis Group
NEW YORK LONDON

First published 2013
by Routledge
711 Third Avenue, New York, NY 10017

Simultaneously published in the UK
by Routledge
2 Park Square, Milton Park, Abingdon, Oxon OX14 4RN

*Routledge is an imprint of the Taylor & Francis Group, an informa business*



*Library of Congress Cataloging-in-Publication Data*

Hughes Rinker, Cortney.
Islam, development, and urban women's reproductive practices / by Cortney Hughes Rinker.
pages cm. — (Routledge studies in anthropology ; 9)
Includes bibliographical references and index.
1. Human reproduction—Government policy—Morocco. 2. Human reproduction—Religious aspects—Islam. 3. Urban women—Morocco. 4. Women—Health and hygiene—Morocco. I. Title.
QP251.H796 2013
612.60964—dc23
2012042914

ISBN13: 978-0-415-81887-2 (hbk)
ISBN13: 978-0-203-38775-7 (ebk)

Typeset in Sabon
by IBT Global.

**To all the women in Morocco who opened up my eyes**

**and**

**To our little one who has taught me what it means to be a mother**

**“The one who wants honey must tolerate bee stings.”**
***l-li bġa l-‘sl y-ṣbr l qris n-nhl.***
**Moroccan Proverb**

# Contents

# Figures and Tables

## FIGURES



## TABLES

# Note on Translation

When appropriate, I have provided English translations of Moroccan Arabic (*darija*), Modern Standard Arabic (*fuṣḥa*), and French words and sentences. I have translated and transliterated terms and phrases in the Moroccan dialect of Arabic to the best of my ability, consulting texts such as *A Basic Course in Moroccan Arabic* (2006) by Richard S. Harrell, Mohammed Abu-Talib, and William S. Carroll and the Peace Corps instruction book on Moroccan Arabic. For any Modern Standard Arabic, I used the *International Journal of Middle East Studies* (IJMES) transliteration system for proper spelling and formatting. My teachers at Al Akhawayn University in Morocco told me that one of the main differences between Moroccan Arabic and Modern Standard Arabic is the absence of long vowels in the Moroccan dialect, although verb conjugations, prepositions, and vocabularies differ as well. Moroccan Arabic has words from French and Spanish as well as from Amazigh dialects. In addition, all French translations are my own. I take complete and full responsibility for any misinterpretation or mistranslation.

# Acknowledgments

This ethnography was only made possible through the love, help, and support of many different individuals. I am forever indebted to more people than I can name in these few pages, and I apologize in advance to anyone whose name I was not able to include here.

I am grateful to my advisor in graduate school, Susan Greenhalgh, for her guidance. I am thankful for the hours she spent reading every word of my papers, proposals, and chapters and for her patience as I tried to turn my data and ideas into something coherent and concise. Her mentorship is more than I could have ever asked for in a dissertation advisor. Victoria Bernal, who as one of my first-year advisors at the University of California Irvine encouraged me to explore feminist theory and research from the very beginning. Mei Zhan introduced me to the world of Science and Technology Studies and to medical anthropology in the anthropology department's first-year graduate seminar and her course Other Knowledges. Lara Deeb offered tremendous insight as to how I can position myself as a Middle East anthropologist. I must sincerely thank them for their critical reading of drafts and for their comments that pushed my thinking and writing. Kaushik Sunder Rajan provided helpful commentary on my dissertation prospectus that I continuously drew upon while conducing fieldwork for this project. Tom Boellstorff, Mike Burton, Teresa Caldeira, Karen Leonard, Bill Maurer, and Jennifer Terry offered a space for me to develop my intellectual voice in their seminars. Conversations with Angela Garcia, Kavita Philip, and Jeanne Scheper at various points in time helped shaped parts of my analysis. Michael Montoya encouraged me to "stay in the place of uncertainty longer" while thinking and writing. I thank Kristin Peterson for taking me on as a research assistant in 2009; the opportunity made me realize the importance of bringing global health and anthropology together to address disparities from the ground up.

My graduate cohort in the Department of Anthropology at UC Irvine, Asya Anderson, Yoon Choi, Jeff Katcherian, and Connie McGuire, made the time go by quickly. I am grateful for having the opportunity to read and struggle with the work of scholars like Marx, Levi-Strauss, Foucault, Agamben, and Gramsci with them. In addition to being an amazing researcher, teacher, and colleague, my cohort member Sheena Nahm provided much needed emotional support. Nanao Akanuma, Erin Moran, Allison Fish, Seo Young Park, and Erica Vogel offered close yet generous readings of my work as well as friendship. Andrea Ballestero, Phillip Grant, Guillermo Navarez, and Robert Werth provided thoughtful suggestions on chapter drafts during our dissertation writing seminars that I took under serious consideration in making revisions. I would like to thank my fellow faculty members in the Department of Sociology and Anthropology at George Mason University, who pushed and supported me through writing this book and made sure I met my deadlines, particularly Andrew Bickford, Rutledge Dennis, Dae Young Kim, Jeff Mantz, Joe Scimecca, Linda Seligmann, and Susan Trencher. I want to also thank graduate students Kim Lufkin, Sara Moore, John Lunsford, and Tara Sheron for conversations that encouraged me to think through tough issues while writing this book. My undergraduate research assistants at George Mason, Oliver Pelland and Serena Abdallah, were gracious enough to help me put the finishing touches on this manuscript.

I have been fortunate enough to receive financial support from various institutions for this work. Long-term research for this project from 2008 to 2009 was supported by grants from the American Institute for Maghrib Studies and the American Philosophical Society. The School of Social Sciences and the Department of Anthropology at UC Irvine funded preliminary fieldwork in Rabat in the summers of 2005, 2006, and 2007. I am thankful to have received the school's pre-dissertation fellowship quarter in the fall of 2007 to prepare for my move to Morocco a few months later. The School of Humanities and Social Sciences at Al Akhawayn University in Ifrane, Morocco, allowed me to be in residence as an affiliate researcher in the fall of 2008. Several faculty members who work on women's issues and development in Morocco offered keen insight as to my work, and I learned a great deal from participating in the university's campus events and interacting with undergraduate and graduate students. Several small portions of this ethnography were presented at academic conferences, including various events at UC Irvine (The CalIT2 Conference, What Is So Hard about Soft Law?, and the brown-bag lunch series in the Department of Women's Studies) in addition to the State of Neoliberalism Graduate Student Conference at the Central European University in Budapest, Hungary, in 2007; the 2008 Middle East Studies Association annual meeting in Washington, DC; the Thinking Gender and State of the Art Conferences at UCLA in 2010; and the 2011 American Anthropological Association annual meeting in Montreal. I thank the organizers for giving me the opportunities to participate and the scholars and community members who provided feedback on these papers, which eventually turned into parts of chapters. I am extremely grateful to Max Novick at Routledge, who saw potential in this book project and gave me a chance to publish it. I also want to thank the wonderful production staff at the press for making this text possible and to

Michael Watters at IBT Global. Portions of Chapters 1, 4, and 5 appear in Medical Anthropology Quarterly 25(4): 417-435. Parts of the prologue and Chapter 2 appear in *Anthropology of the Middle East and North Africa: Into the New Millennium* (Bloomington: Indiana University Press, 2013), edited by Sherine Hafez and Susan Slyomovics. And, portions of Chapters 1, 4, and the conclusion appear in the *Arab Studies Journal* 21(1), spring 2013.

Many friends and family were also present behind the scenes of the fieldwork, data analysis, and writing. My parents, Ron Hughes and Cindy Bohm, have been the greatest support that I could ask for. They provided amazing guidance at critical and opportune times. My father always put his needs second to my own, and my mother offered wisdom when I needed it. My three older brothers, Aaron Hughes, Darrell Hughes, and Chris Salvatore, have always been positive role models in my life, even though they may not have known that I always looked up to them. I could not have gotten through years of fieldwork and writing without friends not listed here. Kelly Damiano Le never ceased her enthusiasm about my work. Notes and emails from Rita Anderson and Maggie Stanton always kept me smiling. Brian Lauri opened up his home to me on trips back to Irvine from Morocco. And last but certainly not least, I must thank my husband, Justin Rinker, for all of his encouragement during this long process. He always believed in me and there was never a day that I did not feel his love and support. He calmed me when I was in a panic and gave me strength when I wanted to give up. This book is dedicated to our little one, who has taught us that a big part of parenthood is putting someone else first and loving that person more than you ever thought was possible.

I must say that I am truly grateful to all of those who took me under their wings and opened up their lives to me during my fieldwork in Morocco. I do not want to identify some of them by their real names so as to preserve their anonymity. I will use pseudonyms here, but I hope they will recognize themselves when they read this: to Hajjer, Meryem, Malika, Noor, Amin, Mr. Masjeel, and Mr. Benbella at the RHO's main office, who opened the doors for me in Morocco; to Fatima, Kaoutar, and Malika, who patiently answered all of my questions with enthusiasm and allowed me to follow them throughout the clinics on a near-daily basis; to the doctors at the hospitals and the clinics (Dr. Senah, Dr. Kinjalli, Dr. Mamouri, Dr. Beni, and Dr. Looz) who allowed me to quietly observe their work; to the interns at the clinics who also allowed me to observe and ask them questions; to Dr. Mohammed, who provided me contacts in the world of Public Health in Morocco and offered critical feedback on my research; to Nora and Haneez, who allowed me to participate in the sewing classes at the health clinic; to Debla and Boutaina, who kept me up-to-date on critical issues in Morocco concerning women's rights and opened up to me about their work over coffee or ice cream every week; to Dr. Binjal, who took the time to meet with me to discuss his experiences working in reproductive healthcare in Morocco and abroad; to Mr. Benjalli and Mrs. Sahali who provided me with resources and information about literacy programs; to Andrew and Diva for being the two best roommates in the world and for helping me think through problems during my fieldwork; to Hind for always having a smile on her face that made me want to smile, too; to Charis, Kris, Elena, Addie, Meredith, Azhar, and Martin, who provided me inspiration and friendship; to Mrs. Abdellah and Mrs. Jones, who sat down with me to provide thoughtful insight; to Mrs. Fisher, Dr. Smith, and Dr. Jayes at Al Akhawayn University, who helped me open up new yet critical questions that needed to be addressed in my work; to Dr. Dahbi, the former Dean of Humanities and Social Sciences, for allowing me to be an affiliate researcher at AUI; to Farida, Misty, Karen, Kevin, Julie, Gerald, and Caroline who made Ifrane feel like my second home for a few months; to Dinar for always making me laugh, mostly unintentionally, and for being patient with my sometimes naive questions about Islam; and to Sarah, Amina, Nawal, Kenza, Saouda, Layla, Ghizlane, Salima, Hadal, Meryem, Habiba, Amal, Nadah, Cherifa, Jahira, Najal, and so many others who welcomed me into their lives and homes. I am very thankful to the communities of Tarma and Zitounia. I hope that everyone who participated in my research will be happy with the results and what I have written in this book.

# Prologue

This ethnography is a study of childbearing and childrearing practices among working-class women living in or near the capital city of Morocco, Rabat. The anthropology of reproduction has often focused on the individual, providing rich detail about the social, cultural, and psychological forces that impact men and women's decision making when it comes to fertility, infertility, medical technologies, childbirth, and contraception. This study builds on work in feminist scholarship and medical anthropology that links individual reproductive practices to broader national and international discourses of development, religion, and health. In trying to discern how the Moroccan government, development organizations, and medical professionals are producing modern reproductive subjects through new development initiatives and reproductive practices, I argue that women appropriate practices and spaces of intervention and turn them into something unrecognizable from the intended purposes. However, at the same time, women also participate in the development agenda that prescribes them as citizens through their very ability to give birth and to control the population.

The main sites for this study are a public health clinic run by the Ministry of Health and two private clinics run by the Reproductive Health Organization (RHO) in Tarma, a suburb of Rabat, and Zitounia, a working-class quarter.[1] Over the course of my research, I spent time in selected female patients' homes and with the RHO community outreach program, too, and I include data from them in this book, but the health clinics are the sites where I could learn the most about modern childbearing and childrearing practices and are the primary focus of my study. The RHO is deeply entrenched in a transnational network of reproductive healthcare and is an officially recognized nongovernmental organization (NGO). The executive staff as well as the clinical staff collaborates with the Ministry of Health in order to provide exceptional care to patients given the available resources. The chief of maternity and obstetrics at a public hospital, Dr. Mamouri, explained to me that the Moroccan government allots only 5 percent of its budget to healthcare, which means organizations like the RHO that sustain themselves through private funding and patients' fees play a crucial role in providing services and care that smaller public health facilities cannot, because the services rendered are free of charge. Conducting fieldwork in these clinics allowed me to examine the processes by which reproductive practices circulated between international, national, and individual levels within their social context.

My decision to conduct research primarily in the health clinics, women's homes, and the local communities was not easy and offered some problems that I would not have encountered if I chose to only work in the main offices of the Ministry of Health, the RHO, or development agencies in Rabat. I start here with how I came to study reproduction in Morocco and within these particular sites and then move on to a discussion of some of the issues I faced during fieldwork. This prologue focuses on how the clinics and women's homes are specific sites of institutional intervention (as well as resistance) and also offers insight into my position as an anthropologist conducting research in medical facilities in North Africa.

In 2005, when research for this ethnographic project very first began, I was studying Moroccan Arabic in Fes, Morocco (located about two hours east of Rabat), and I continued my studies of the dialect and French over the next few years in the country and in the United States. I had studied Arabic in Morocco as an undergraduate and was now returning for preliminary fieldwork as a graduate student. As part of a tourist excursion one weekend, I traveled with twenty other American students to the outskirts of the Sahara for a weekend camping trip. We slept in tents in an oasis that could only be reached by riding a camel from the town for two hours. I woke up suddenly in the middle of the night to excruciating pain in my shoulder and was rushed to the local medical clinic via a four-by-four vehicle as soon as the sun came up along with a middle-aged South African woman, Jane, who was our supervisor. The doctor was not at the clinic; he had to be picked up from his nearby home by our guides. Once he arrived, he unlocked the door and led us into the clinic. It was small and bare with only an office, an exam room, and a waiting room. We followed him into the exam room. On the door was a poster advertising oral contraception. It pictured a family comprised of a mother and father and two children, a boy and a girl. They were smiling and dressed in T-shirts and pants while standing against a white background. Jane saw the poster, too, and said under her breath, "I wonder what is his practice like? Starving children? Stung tourists? Look at this place. And then this poster is in the clinic?"

Whereas this experience for me was my first look at reproductive health in Morocco, it also provided a window into how reproduction was being integrated into the public health system and how women's reproductive bodies, and in particular working-class bodies, were being incorporated into discourses surrounding modernization and health. Given this, the objective of my remaining preliminary research trips in the summers of 2006 and 2007, and my long-term study from January 2008 to July 2009, was to see how the development agenda in Morocco was filtered through reproductive practices both inside and outside of clinics and how women understood and utilized such practices in their daily lives. Morocco held elections in late 2011 and the Islamist party won the most seats in Parliament. I conducted research at the time when the *Istiqlāl* party (*Ḥizb al-Istiqlāl* in Arabic, or *Parti de l'Istiqlal* in French), a conservative party, was in power, so I recognize that this ethnography may look very different if I had conducted research after the latest election.

In 2006, my preliminary work included an internship at the main office of the RHO. I discussed with Mr. Masjeel, the executive director, my role as an intern and a researcher and the possibility of returning to conduct even further research in the health clinics in the future. At that time, my main role was to help construct a patient satisfaction survey through making observations and speaking with staff (counselors and doctors) in the nearby RHO health clinics. I worked primarily in the Tarma clinic, which provided me easy access to the public health center because it was right next door. When I returned to the RHO in early 2008, Mr. Masjeel was more than willing to allow me to intern again so that I could conduct further observations and interviews in the clinics as well as with executive staff members, clinical staff, and participants in the community outreach program. My connection with the RHO proved fruitful in that it gave me legitimacy as a researcher of reproductive health and allowed me to make contacts somewhat effortlessly within the Ministry of Health, public health clinics and hospitals, and national and international development agencies.

Although having the title of *stagiaire* (intern) at the RHO was certainly beneficial to my research purposes, it also proved to be hindering at some points. I never worked under direct supervision at the main office of the RHO, but rather was given rein to pick and choose the projects I wanted to participate in, such as helping translate documents from French to English and vice versa or helping coordinate the annual youth festival. The executive staff members, however, were very much aware of my desire to be in the clinics as much as possible, and I was one of a few individuals who were not part of the medical staff who would be there (representatives from international aid agencies, pharmaceutical reps, other researchers, etc.). I knew however, that I would be spending considerably more time in the clinics than most others. One constraint that I faced while conducting research outside of the main RHO office was my position as an intern. My loyalty was tested on several occasions. The executive staff did not travel frequently to the clinics, and the clinical staff only attended a few meetings at the main office. Although there is a regional coordinator for the clinics, she could not visit each of the six clinics in the Rabat region every day. (She left the RHO about half way through my fieldwork, and the position was not filled as my fieldwork came to an end.) One day I was watching a video at the main office produced by the RHO about the community outreach program. I watched the man, Amin, who I traveled with several times during my preliminary work in particular on the screen. Part of the film documented his work with the RHO volunteers, who would purchase birth control pills and condoms from him and then sell them to men and women in their local areas. The staff member who showed me this film asked me, "Is that what he does?" He wanted to know if Amin actually carried out the practices he showed on the film during his outreach trips, which took place one or two days a week. This question made me reasonably uncomfortable because this staff member wanted me to use my research experience to state matter-of-factly whether or not Amin was doing his job. Whereas this incident was an extreme case, some of the executive staff members demanded answers from me about why poorer Moroccan women tended to have larger families or how they could improve the care the patients received. I felt as though my interviews and observations in the clinics could possibly be used against the medical staff who made my research possible, which made me be extremely careful about how I collected data and how I recorded my observations and interviews.

Even though I was generally comfortable working with the medical staff, I was still concerned that I did not make the female patients feel as though they were required to speak to me in order to receive care, whether that might be from my presence in the counseling room, my conversations with them in the waiting rooms, or my note taking during their visits with the doctor. The doctors I worked with were more than happy to have me observe their work, but both of us always asked the female patient prior to the start of their examinations. The counselors, on the other hand, were eager to have me speak to the women who attended the clinics and would sometimes insist that I speak to them in the waiting rooms—to the point that I had to refrain from attending the clinics for two weeks during the beginning of my fieldwork until I spoke with the executive staff. This made the atmosphere very uncomfortable for me and for the female patients I was being forced upon. Once it was clear that I needed time to introduce myself and to make the patients aware of my purposes, I returned to the clinics. However, given that I was not a medical student and do not have medical training, it was not appropriate for me to be present in the exam room for female patients' annual gynecological exams or any medically invasive procedures. I was permitted to observe the interactions between patients and the doctors prior to and after, but not during. This ethnography focuses on consultations between clinical staff and patients, interactions between female patients themselves, and my conversations and observations.

My identity as an American anthropologist was both beneficial and constraining to my research. In the clinics, female patients often did not understand what I did when I explained it to them and assumed that I was training to become a medical doctor. They would often ask me for medical advice, which I could not prescribe. All I could do was refer them to a member of the clinical staff who could. There were many times when my training as social scientist, instead of as a physician or in another biological science, was valuable because it allowed me to ask medical practitioners and patients for descriptions of practices and then I could compare the two. For example, I asked one female patient in the waiting room about her use of the birth control pill. She responded, "I don't want to use it. Look at my face; there are spots! These are from the pill." The three obstetrician gynecologists (OB/GYNs) I worked with on a regular basis at the RHO clinics consistently explained that these spots were not from the pill but, rather, from the hormone changes that come with pregnancy. Similarly, being an American and a non-Muslim provided me with numerous opportunities to ask questions about cultural and religious beliefs and practices that "native observers" could not. For instance, I could comfortably ask individuals to tell me what they understand Islam to say about contraception, pregnancy, motherhood, and health or about the hierarchy of power within the household.

However, at the same time, my identity as an American became somewhat of an impediment when I moved my research out of the clinics and into female patients' homes, mainly during the last seven months of my fieldwork in 2009. It is common knowledge in Morocco that receiving a visa to the United States or Europe can be extremely difficult due to the criteria that needs to be met. Moroccans must prove that they have ties in Morocco that will cause them to return, such as work obligations, property, or a bank account. One way to surpass this, especially for working and lower-middle-class individuals who do not have financial resources, is by marrying an American or European citizen, although there is no guarantee as to when the visa will be issued. A friend of mine who worked for a European embassy stated that she would delay issuing the visa for as long as possible if she believed the marriage might be forced, fake, or for profit.[2] I found this within my own work. Sometimes I questioned whether the female patients from the clinics allowed me into their homes because they were interested in my work, or because they intended for me to marry their brother, cousin, or other male relative in order for him to get a visa. There was a thin line between researcher and potential bride that I had to tread. I had worked closely with a staff member at the RHO, Omama, for six months before she asked me at a café one afternoon over lunch, "When will you convert to Islam so you can marry my brother? He really wants to go to the United States." I was definitely not prepared for this question and was almost speechless after she finished asking. Similarly, I had visited Amal, a female patient from the clinic in Zitounia, in her home several times before her husband told me, "You can travel the world, but you come back to Morocco to get married." I asked, "Who will I marry?" Amal looked at me and said, "Mohammed of course!" Mohammed was her older brother who dreamed of moving to the United States for work, even though he did not have his high school diploma. He left school when he was about fourteen years old and worked odd jobs here and there to make ends meet. It was only a few days later that Mohammed began calling me day and night, leaving me no choice but to end my work with Amal and her family. (In an attempt to avoid this type of situation, I explained numerous times to men and women alike that I had a partner in the United States and was not willing to marry in Morocco.) Being an American researcher at times allowed me better access to female patients in their homes, which enabled me to examine how women appropriate the reproductive practices in the clinics within their daily lives, but due to the bureaucratic structures in Morocco and the relatively high unemployment rate, it also made it difficult at times to maintain professional relationships with female patients outside of the clinics.

These issues and my position and identity informed the types of questions I could ask, the people I could speak with, and the places that I could go while conducting research, and I am cognizant of this throughout my analysis. I turned to feminist scholarship when I had to grapple with several methodological questions throughout my research and the process of writing (Harding 1987, 2004; Kum-kum 2004). How could my work possibly benefit the female patients, medical providers, government officials, and development workers who participated? How could I negotiate my own position within the homes and families that I visited? How could I write about female patients and Moroccan women in nongeneralizable ways? How could I attribute agency and power to them in my work? I empathized with patients. Sometimes I cried with them, and at other times I became angry just like they were. I had to learn how to reel these emotions in and how to deal with them during fieldwork and the writing process. Rayna Rapp, in her study of amniocentesis in New York City, posits that "the ethics of fieldwork must include a constant assessment of the limited benefits and possible harm researchers can do, in situations where racial, ethnic, national, and religious stereotypes are built into communicative and social service interactions across class differences" (2000, 22). For me, these assessments are never ending and have impacted my research and writing practices, such as not tape-recording informal conversations with patients and clinical staff and trying to portray as accurately as I can Moroccan women's experiences and how they talked about responsibility, control, the future, their bodies, reproduction, and health.

The goal of this book, however, is not just to address methodological questions about conducting research in medical settings, in intimate places like the home, and in larger bureaucratic organizations. It is also to problematize theoretical debates concerning reproduction, gender, development, and religion taking place in anthropology and across disciplines. A large part of this project is to situate Morocco within the Middle East and North Africa and on the global stage through an in-depth analysis of childbearing and childrearing practices. For instance, one afternoon I was walking with Salima from the RHO health clinic after she had a *contrôle*, or follow-up visit, for her intrauterine device (IUD). After she asked what I thought of Morocco, and I responded, she stated that she loved the country even though she had family living abroad in Europe. I inquired why she liked the country so much. She explained, "Because it's not France. It's not Europe, but it's not Saudi Arabia. It's *Islamique*." Salima continued, "It's Islamic but we can do these things here. It's not haram [forbidden]." Here the words "things" and "this" referred to contraception. Salima used contraceptive methods as a way to position Morocco within the Middle East region and to frame the geopolitical context of Islam.

Just as Morocco adapts and shapes international discourses surrounding women's bodies, fertility, and human rights, I constantly link everyday and mundane practices to broader contexts. By locating reproductive practices—medical and nonmedical in nature—that some women and medical providers have come to see as routine whereas others view them as contested, I aim to show how women, doctors, the government, and development agencies negotiate discourses as they create new meanings of modern citizenship that must keep up with a rapidly transitioning Morocco.

# Introduction

## Building Modern Morocco One Woman at a Time

Several feminist scholars have argued that women's bodies are important sites by which political and cultural transitions are carried out and results are gauged. Victoria Bernal stresses "gender plays a significant role in the intersection of global and local cultures" (1997, 131). More importantly, feminist research has demonstrated that reproduction has a critical role in how a nation defines and imagines itself. Faye Ginsburg and Rayna Rapp, in their landmark text *Conceiving the New World Order: The Global Politics of Reproduction*, claim that in its "biological and social senses" reproduction is "inextricably bound up with the production of culture" (1995, 2). Nira Yuval-Davis writes, "The central importance of women's reproductive roles in ethnic and national discourses becomes apparent when one considers that one usually joins the collectivity by being born into it" (2001, 123). Such scholars have forcefully critiqued theories of nationalism and citizenship in a rapidly globalizing world that have left out questions of gender and reproduction (cf. Anderson 1991; Gellner 1983; Smith 1995). In Morocco, reproduction is central to the state's recent development policies and plays a critical role in the ways that women are framed as citizens. A development report for the country, *50 Ans de Développement Humain et Perspectives 2025* (50 Years of Human Development and Prospects to 2025) even reads, "Thanks to the changes in matrimonial and procreative behaviors of Moroccan women. . . . and family planning programs in which a large portion of the female population participated, the country was able to manage the development of its population" (Royume du Maroc 2006, 8). Building on feminist critiques, this ethnography examines how women's reproductive and childrearing practices and their reproductive bodies have become integral to development programs in Morocco and distills the ways women interpret such practices and see themselves as becoming modern citizens.

Defining modern citizenship in Morocco today is not an easy task given the country is undergoing rapid social and economic development. So to not essentialize the concept and to allow the contestations and contradictions to emerge, I focus on the practices and discourses of modern citizenship within the Moroccan context. In entering theoretical debates about gender, citizenship, and Islam in the Middle East and North Africa (MENA), this ethnography brings a different perspective because it tells the story of modernization through reproductive practices. In scholarship on the MENA, Morocco, along with other parts of the Maghrib including Algeria, Tunisia, and Libya, is often an outlier because of its geographical positioning and French colonial history. Edmund Burke argues Morocco and the Maghrib inhabit an ambiguous space that is "not quite Africa, not quite Arab, not quite European" (2000, 17). Although there has been a good amount of social science research conducted in the country by Moroccan and foreign scholars alike, its constant political, cultural, and economic transitions have produced new questions to be asked and new topics to be covered. Part of this ethnographic project is to demonstrate Morocco's complicated location within the MENA and within global discourses of reproductive health and development through a discussion of childbearing and childrearing practices among working-class urban women.

In popular culture, images of Morocco have usually evoked feelings of mystery, enchantment, and delight (Rabinow 1977; Waugh 2005). It is marked as part of the Orient, and Edward Said emphasizes that "neither the term Orient nor the concept of the West has any ontological stability; each is made up of human effort, partly affirmation, partly identification with the Other" (1979, xvii). Morocco's location on the continent of Africa just miles from Spain in combination with its deep ties to the Middle East through its Arab and Muslim populations and adoption of the Arabic language has posed challenges to the borders of "East" and "West." The March 2010 issue of the popular *Delta Sky Magazine*, which I found in the seat pocket in front of me on a flight from Detroit to Santa Ana, California, featured an article on Morocco. It quoted the country's late King Hassan II (c. 1929–1999) as stating that Morocco is a "tree, the roots of which are planted firmly in Africa but has its branches in Europe."[1] Paul Silverstein notes the Moroccan government has faced "ethnic, racial, and religious fragmentation from within and political-demographic pressures from without" (2005, 27). Silverstein argues that these internal and external pressures are linked as the country's increased economic relationships with Europe and the United States are partially based upon its ability to control religious fundamentalism and Islamic groups. He suggests that a "fractured . . . landscape thus persists as the ground on which the contemporary North African politics . . . take place" (ibid.).

In August 2009, an article in the *New York Times* entitled "Islamic Radicalism Slows Moroccan Reforms" describes Morocco as the "rare liberalizing, modernizing Islamic state, open to the West and a potential bridge to a calmer Middle East that can live in peace with Israel" (Erlanger and Mekhennet 2009). However, the article states pressure, particularly from Islamic radicalism in the country, has hindered the seemingly rapid pace of change. The November 2011 win of the PJD, or Justice and Development Party (*Parti de la justice et du développement*), has raised further concern among international organizations (IOs) and governments about the role of Islam in policy making. The PJD is a moderate Islamist party from which the new prime minister, Abdelilah Benkirane, was appointed. The party does not describe itself as an "Islamist" party per se, but rather as having an Islamic reference, meaning that its policies follow the moral dictates of the religion. It has been hailed as one of the most modern and democratic parties in Morocco (Liddell 2008). The PJD "focused first on social issues, such as opposition to summer music festivals and the sale of alcohol, but has shifted to issues with broader voter appeal like the fight against corruption and high unemployment" (Al Arabiya and Agencies 2011). The party will promote Islamic finance, but it has not focused on issues such as headscarves for women given that Morocco attracts a large number of Western tourists (Hamilton 2011). State officials are concerned with keeping a proper balance between "freedom and social cohesion." When I made my first trip to Morocco in late May of 2003 as an undergraduate, the country was recovering from the worst bombing in its history, which took place in Casablanca just weeks prior to my arrival. Suicide bombers from Salafia Jihadia, a group with supposed connections to Al Qaeda, killed forty-eight civilians when they attacked foreign establishments in the city center.[2] Since this event and a thwarted attack in 2007, there has been a crackdown on Islamic and oppositional groups and closer monitoring of mosques by the order of King Mohammed VI, who took the throne in 1999. The king believes himself to be a reformer, according to the *New York Times* article, "having invested heavily in economic development, loosened restraints on the news media, given more rights to women and shed light on some of the worst human-rights abuses of the past" (Erlanger and Mekhennet 2009). However, to not ignite more conservative views of Islam and political organizations, the king has slowed reform, in particular of laws governing women's rights.

Mr. Fouad Ali El Himma, a former deputy interior minister and leader of the Authenticity and Modernity Party (PAM) in Morocco, has spoken fervently about reform in the country. He has stated, "Morocco 'has always been a country of transit'" (quoted in Erlanger and Mekhennet 2009). How are reproduction and women's reproductive bodies central to this time of transition in Morocco? What roles do women play in reform? How do their practices of childbearing and childrearing adhere to, contradict, or create new notions of modern citizenship? The premise of this ethnography is the transition from economic development to social development that began to take shape during the mid to late 1990s in Morocco. In 2005, King Mohammed VI launched the National Initiative for Human Development *(l'Initiative nationale pour le développement humain* or INDH), an important social policy that makes improving citizens' lives the top political priority. After years of focusing on economic growth with the belief that financial gains would improve social indicators (illiteracy, healthcare, education, poverty) the government shifted its attention to human development, a move that engaged with global changes in development rhetoric (Rose 1999). The king has emphasized to the Parliament and the nation that development is hinged upon the country's citizens, and, for this reason, it is the duty of the state to foster a new mentality in men and women that concentrates on "entrepreneurship, participation, and production" (Ben-Meir 2005). In short, they must be prepared to make responsible decisions about their lives—such as having smaller families—and to become "modernized" citizens.

Anthropologists and feminist scholars in particular have argued that development programs tend to be "gender-blind" or ignore the differential impacts on men and women (Clarke 2006; Hodgson 2001; Parpart et al. 2000; Smith and Cohen 2000). This ethnography provides a bridge between conceptualizations of development and alternative modernities and feminist accounts of reproduction. Reproduction, I argue, provides a very valuable case study to understand how feminine citizenship is being constructed and enabled in Morocco within policies and everyday practices given the sometimes contradicting cultural, religious, and political discourses. Reproduction and development are both "forward-looking," as women bring children into this world who will become the future citizens. Jennifer Johnson-Hanks (2006a), in her comparative study of Muslim and non-Muslim fertility in West Africa, suggests that since September 11, 2001, Muslim women have been viewed as overreproductive in both academic and popular discourses, but with a close examination, she demonstrates that birth rates are dependent upon social context, not religion. By putting working-class Moroccan women's lives at the center of this ethnography, I am able to challenge this connection between Islam, poverty, and fertility while delineating the complicated ways that women are incorporated into development and constructed as citizens.

I am not suggesting that reproduction has not been an issue in Morocco for a period of time; in fact, it has been a lingering concern since the decades following independence from France in 1956. Although the Total Fertility Rate (TFR) has dramatically decreased from 7.4 children per woman in 1973 (Courbage 1995) to 2.3 children today, the annual population growth rate remains relatively high (1.4%) and approximately one-third of the total population is under the age of fifteen.[3] Given these statistics, reproduction has come to be seen as a foundation for development in Morocco—if the population growth is not controlled, then there may not be enough academic and professional opportunities for children as they become older, thus hindering the country's role in the global economic and political stage.

*Table I.1* The TFR for Morocco

| Year | Total Fertility Rate |
|---|---|
| 1980 | 5.6 |
| 1985 | 4.9 |
| 1990 | 4.0 |
| 1995 | 3.3 |
| 2000 | 2.7 |
| 2004 | 2.4 |
| 2010 | 2.3 |

*Source:* Adapted from the World Bank, "Fertility Rate (Total Births per Woman)"[4]

This ethnography is based upon my three main research questions: What are the reproductive subjects that the government is attempting to create through new initiatives, in particular the INDH? What are the childbearing and childrearing practices associated with these subjects? And, finally, how do working-class women interpret these practices and how do they impact how they see themselves as modern citizens? In an attempt to sketch out the answers, I argue that the working-class and middle-class women appropriate practices and spaces of reproductive intervention—clinics, contraception, and ultrasounds, for instance—and make them nearly unrecognizable in comparison to how the state and development organizations intended them to be. At the same time, these women participate unwittingly in the development agenda and policies that prescribe them as citizens through their very abilities to control the fertility rate and population growth. In this process, Moroccan women illustrate various representations of modernity as their goals for inhabiting such spaces and using such practices intersect with those of the medical community, governing bodies, and development agencies—smaller families, higher-caliber children, greater use of reproductive healthcare services—but the meanings they give to these spaces and practices vary, which produces new facets of modern neoliberal citizenship as they redefine notions of womanhood and motherhood.

## FIELDWORK IN MOROCCO

Research for this project took place in two primary places: Tarma and Zitounia. To protect the anonymity of participants, I have fictionalized the places' names and will not disclose their exact locations in Morocco. I will provide a very general overview about the sites. Tarma is a suburb of the capital city Rabat that is made up of approximately 225,000 people. Tarma is located close to the center of Rabat and Casablanca, which are the political and economic epicenters of the country, respectively. Foreign and domestic corporations have established industries in its surrounding areas, including textile factories, electronics, and chemical plants. In 2006, when I took a trip with a community outreach worker run by the RHO, we drove through Tarma and I noticed several women, all dressed in blue and white, lining picnic tables along the road eating lunch. When I asked the driver what these women were doing, he stated that they worked in the factory that produces watches nearby. An Italian company owned the factory. Tarma has not only become a hub for potential tourist activity, but is also becoming a popular location for international and domestically run factories given its proximity to Rabat and Casablanca and relatively large population of inexpensive labor.[5]

Whereas the elite of Morocco flock to the coastal areas of Tarma, the neighborhoods located further inland are working class, lined with vegetable and fruit stands, butcher shops, and inexpensive clothing stores. These areas of Tarma are changing, however. They have been the sites of state-run programs to eradicate shantytowns and to improve living conditions. In 2006, the government designated 3.25 billion dirhams (US$361 million)[6] to a specific project in the region to refurbish roads, increase green spaces, and establish places for social gatherings. In addition, money was dedicated to relocate about four thousand families living in the shantytowns to a new government-subsidized housing development.[7] In Tarma, buildings are being constructed in mass, but many remain empty because people are unable to afford the prices. One of the female patients from the clinics who lives in Tarma told me as we walked through her neighborhood, "Come back in ten years and maybe this will be finished." We were strolling along a road where the public bus travels that still consists of just dirt and sand even after months of construction.

Like Tarma, Zitounia is a primarily working-class quarter located in Rabat. Residents told me, "Do not buy fruits and vegetables in Sidi Hassain. Buy them here in Zitounia. They are much cheaper and better." Sidi Hassain is where I lived; it is the next quarter over and known for its foreign communities, upscale shopping, international food chains, and private schools. Juxtaposed to this, Zitounia is known by some as a poorer and somewhat violent neighborhood. Others know Zitounia for the large number of men and women from sub-Saharan Africa living in the quarter.

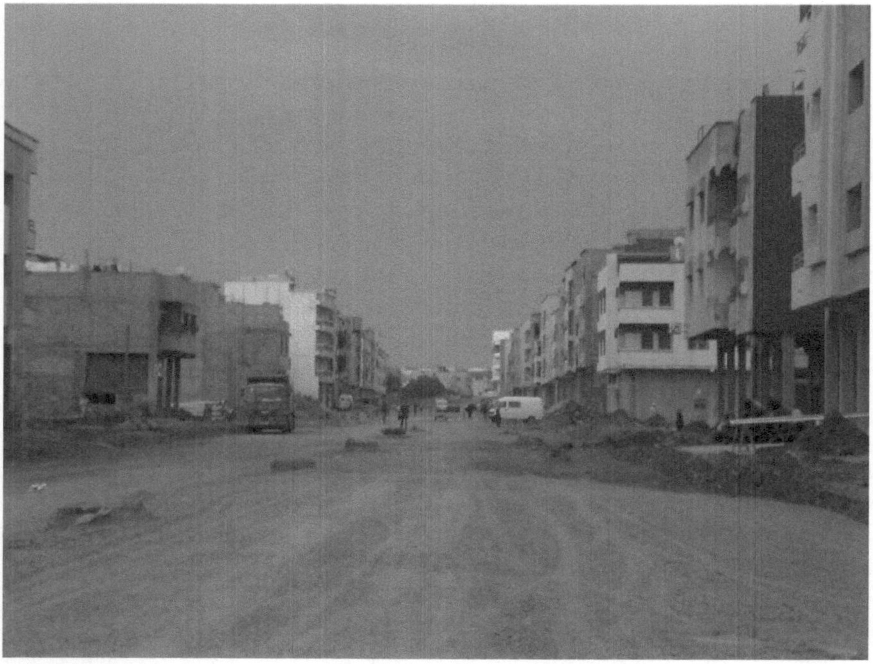

*Figure I.1* An area near Tarma where development of new housing is taking place. (Photo by the author)

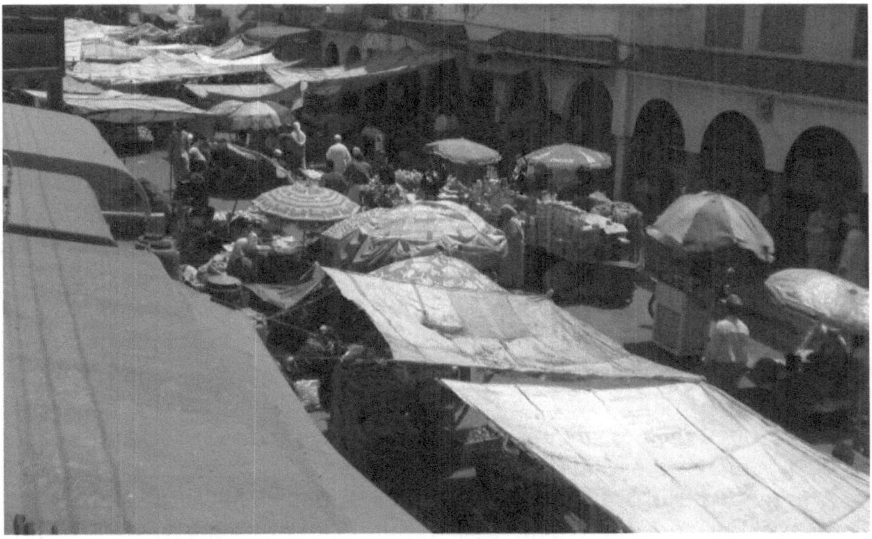

*Figure I.2* A main street in Zitounia. (Photo by the author)

The rent was much less expensive than other parts of Rabat, albeit the buildings were not in the best condition, but this made it much easier for people from countries such as Ghana or Nigeria to find housing as they settled in Morocco or tried to make their way to Europe either legally or illegally. Zitounia is a self-built neighborhood that was established after independence in 1956. The newly independent state required a massive number of civil servants in the capital. People from the rural areas flocked to Rabat, but the housing market was unable to keep up. Zitounia was one of the quarters where such workers set up their homes. Rabat encompasses major extremes. Streets lined with expensive villas next to crowded *bidonvilles*. Zitounia is one of these working-class areas. In the middle of the quarter, next to several elementary and middle schools, sits the main mosque. On Friday afternoons, men line the inside of the mosque, and many bring their prayer rugs to sit outside in the streets to pray and to listen.

## RESEARCH IN THE CLINICS

I would like to begin my discussion of childbearing and childrearing practices by taking the audience through a usual day of fieldwork in Rabat. In this section, I will give a general overview of the events and conversations I had with various individuals that occurred on different occasions. In later chapters of this book, I will give more thorough descriptions of the medical encounters between patients and providers and my interviews with different individuals. I will take a moment here to give some background information about the medical providers and their roles in the clinics, although the three main "characters" of this ethnography will be given more attention in this chapter.

One morning during the week, I arrived at the RHO clinic in Tarma at 8:00 a.m., when it opened to the public. It is located off of the main road that runs from Tarma to Rabat and is not difficult to spot from the nearby bus stop. Just like other days, when I entered the waiting room, I noticed women in djellabas[8] crowding around the counseling room waiting to be checked in by Fatima, the clinic's director. I was first formally introduced to her in 2006 when I was interning at the RHO and then again by two executive staff members once I arrived in 2008. On this day, the OB/GYN and the dermatologist were seeing patients in the afternoon. All of the RHO's clinics, including Zitounia, offer additional services, such as dermatology, pediatrics, psychiatry, and general medicine. The former director of programs of the organization explained to me, "This is to keep women coming to the clinics and to increase the number of patients we see." Fatima and Kaoutar, the director of the clinic in Zitounia, required that all patients take a number when they walked through the door and to wait their turn before they entered the counseling room. On this day, Fatima grabbed my hand and escorted me into the counseling room, which was located just off the waiting room and housed her desk, a cupboard for patients' charts, two chairs, a scale, and a small table for her supplies. She asked me to take the women's numbers when they entered the room and to record their weights. I agreed. When women stepped on the scale, I told Fatima their weight in French, as all of the women's charts were recorded in the language. As I did this, many of them asked, "What did she say?" in Moroccan Arabic. I then translated the number for them into the dialect. Even though the main language of healthcare in Morocco is French, a large portion of women the RHO clinics and the public health clinic served did not understand or speak it because they did not attend school.

A good portion of my fieldwork each day took place in the counseling rooms. The Zitounia clinic was much smaller in size than the one in Tarma and was located on the second floor of an apartment building, up a narrow and winding staircase. The counseling room there was much larger than in Tarma, but it had no door to afford women privacy with Kaoutar. There was even a large window that could not be closed, which looked into the waiting room. As women would tell Fatima and Kaoutar why they had come to the clinic, I sat near their desks taking notes. They both asked me on different days, "What are you writing?" I explained I did not have a good memory and needed to document the conversations for my research. They stated, "Like me!" because I was taking notes just as they did in women's charts. Whereas Fatima and Kaoutar could write something in the patients' charts that could impact the doctor's examination or recommendation, I did not have this authority in the clinic. Their question, I believe, also spoke to their concern that I would be giving this information to the staff at the RHO's main office (i.e., their bosses), but I assured them this would not be the case and everything I wrote in my journal would be for my eyes only.

Sometimes I would work directly with the interns at the RHO clinics. The organization had partnerships with several local training programs that specialized in medical professions and offered students rotations in its clinics. The young intern Zena was adamant that I help her administer pregnancy tests one morning at the Zitounia clinic. She was studying to become a nurse. Rapid pregnancy tests were one of the most popular services at the RHO's clinics. The public health clinic did not offer them; therefore, in Tarma, the staff would refer women to the RHO if they thought they could be pregnant. Women were required to bring their own urine sample to the clinic. Zena gathered the samples, marked each one so they would not be confused, and signaled for me to follow her into the exam room. The room was located just off the waiting room. It was small with a window that overlooked a local market. It had a table for gynecological exams and ultrasounds and a desk for the doctor to write his or her notes. Zena set five different test strips, small pieces of plastic with windows for plus or minus signs, on the exam table and then instructed me to take drops of urine from each jar and place it on the strips. I was forced to think of how to respectfully decline given that I had no training to administer pregnancy tests or to give women their results. I asked if I could just watch. She smiled at me and agreed. Fatima typically performed these tests right in her office, and so did Kaoutar. In addition to pregnancy tests, the RHO clinics offered contraception, ultrasounds, OB/GYN consultations, infertility treatments, and testing for sexually transmitted diseases (STDs). The public health clinic, on the other hand, due to its small size, only offered contraception and often told female patients to go to the RHO when they became pregnant. Not only did the RHO rely on local institutions for help staffing the clinics, but it also used its close connections with the Ministry of Health to gain patients.

Fatima and Kaoutar would check patients in every morning, which meant recording needed services in their charts, taking their weight and blood pressure, and accepting payment. Unlike the public health clinic where all services were free, the services at the RHO clinics were subsidized and patients still had to pay a small fee. Doctors did not arrive usually until the late morning or the afternoon. The exam rooms in the Tarma clinic were located down a hallway from the waiting room. The rooms at the Tarma clinic were similar to the one in Zitounia, except there were two of them. One room was used for general practitioners and the dermatologist, and the other was specific to obstetrics and gynecology, with an ultrasound machine and table with stirrups for exams. No major procedures took place at the clinics because of their lack of equipment. Zitounia even had to share its ultrasound machine with four other clinics in the Rabat region. Dr. Senah, an OB/GYN who worked at the military hospital, often let me observe her when she was with patients at Tarma's and Zitounia's clinics. Dr. Senah received her medical training in

Morocco, but she holds her graduate degree from a university in the United States. She has worked at the RHO for ten years, first as a substitute doctor and then as part-time. She now sees patients two days a week there. I would sit with her near the ultrasound machine, and she would walk me through the process. She looked at me one day and said, "This must be like Chinese to you!" As she was performing an ultrasound, she told me about the patient, whom she had seen before:

> She is about seven months pregnant. We are hoping for a girl. She already has a boy at home. I have seen her twice before for ultrasounds and she came to me when she was pregnant for the first time. See, look we measure the baby's head [*performing the calculations on the screen*] and try to find out the weight. Yes, she is having a girl; look here, you can see the lips, is that what they are called in English? I think so. The baby looks healthy, a good size. She will not have to come back to see me before she gives birth, only if she has a problem.

Women are recommended to have three ultrasounds during a pregnancy, once every three months. On some other days when I was able to observe Dr. Senah, I would sit with her near the desk in the room to listen closely to her conversations with patients after her examination was over. I noticed

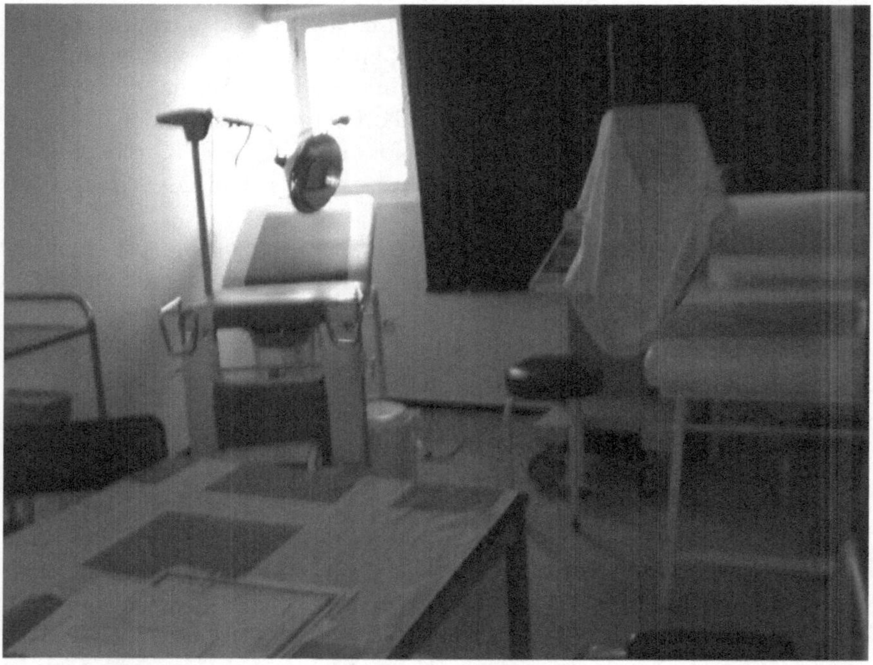

*Figure I.3* The exam room for obstetrics and gynecology. (Photo by the author.)

that Dr. Senah worked quickly given that on certain days, she had to see about thirty female patients in two or three hours. She, like the other doctors and the clinics' directors, never left the clinic until the very last patient was seen, even if it was beyond closing time. The RHO took pride in the quality of care that its medical providers give to patients.

When Zulima came to the RHO clinic in Tarma, she was suffering from a minor stomach virus. Fatima stated the generalist was not in that day and that she should see the doctor at the public health clinic. I walked Zulima over to the clinic, run by the Ministry of Health, just a few yards away. I waited for Zulima to take a number to see the doctor. The public health clinic in Tarma saw as many as fifty or sixty patients each day. The clinic offers basic healthcare, but because specialists are not available, it does not offer reproductive health or maternal health services, except for contraception. The clinic, which I worked in every few weeks when staff offered Maternal and Child Health (SME) sessions, was smaller in size. Zulima took a number from the woman standing in the doorway and found a seat in the already cramped waiting room, located immediately as you entered the doorway. A nurse sat at the desk, just near the entrance, and would distribute medications to patients as they left. Four small exam rooms were off of the waiting room, and there was constant hustle and bustle as patients and staff moved in and out of them. Because this clinic offers various services to all individuals, there was a constant stream of people entering and exiting the relatively small building. The most common problems treated here were colds, stomach viruses, infections, and other basic health problems that could be diagnosed and treated by a general physician. Zulima, who was in her early twenties, waited for nearly thirty minutes before she was called to see the doctor. She emerged with a prescription and then was on her way, leaving behind the other twenty people or so that had come after her to wait their turns.

An additional service offered at the RHO Tarma clinic is a sewing class for women. To the right of the main entry is a specific classroom dedicated to sewing, complete with sewing machines. This is the only sewing class the RHO offers in its clinics in the Rabat region. The women who voluntarily participate must purchase their own fabric and sketchbooks. With the help of two teachers, Nora and Haneez, the women make clothes or household decorations for friends and family or to be sold at the markets. Nora convinced me to try the sewing class, but I was never successful and eventually was "demoted" to runner. From time to time, women in the class would showcase their work at the clinic for the public. People could come to buy the goods. Nora and Haneez instructed these women one-on-one rather than giving a lecture. Nora explained, "Women take this class because it is our culture. They can learn their Moroccan heritage and traditions and make extra money for their families and themselves." Nora emphasized how important this class was for many women as it was sometimes their only way to help their families earn extra income.

Because I was technically an intern at the RHO, I had unlimited access to the various rooms in the clinics. I had little trouble following medical staff during their work day, but of course I respected the times when they needed a little more space, such as in meetings or treating more difficult cases. My presence became normalized as time went on, and the staff and patients were not surprised to see me. Fatima even said to me one afternoon over lunch, "You need to be here tomorrow at 10:00 a.m. The doctor arrives at 11:00 a.m. We have work to do." It was the week of inventory where all of the supplies needed to be counted and a report generated, by hand, for the main office.

## CONDUCTING FORMAL AND INFORMAL INTERVIEWS

What I just recounted is an example of a typical day of participant observation in the health clinics. This is where the majority of my fieldwork took place. I was able to move outside of the clinics and into female patients' homes during the second half of my fieldwork. This was only after I built a strong rapport with several patients and with the staff. Also, I worked from time to time at the RHO headquarters in Rabat, rode along with the community outreach worker for the region, and participated in various events put on by the organization. Many of my later encounters began in the clinics, such as when I was invited to the home of a patient, who then introduced me to another patient or to her extended family members with whom I then worked as well or I tagged along with the outreach worker because he had to take the shared ultrasound machine to another clinic. Whereas my field sites certainly extended beyond the clinics, I found that being able to do work in these other places would not have been possible without the relationships I formed with others inside the facilities.

I also conducted informal interviews with female patients, Fatima, Kaoutar, five doctors (four OB/GYNs and one family practitioner), the director of the public health clinic where I conducted fieldwork, six interns (two from the public health clinic and four from the RHO clinics), and the sewing teachers at the RHO clinic in Tarma. A number of these individuals were interviewed two or three times, but this depended on how often I was able to see them. Sometimes patients who I interviewed would not return to the clinic or would come on a day in which I was not able to be there. Most interviews took place at the clinics and were during normal business hours; this is why I needed to conduct more informal conversations rather than structured interviews. It would not have been possible for the physicians in particular to sit down and speak with me at length, although I was able to do that with one of them at his office at the local hospital, Dr. Mamouri. He allowed me to formally interview him at his office one afternoon in 2008. Many of the physicians were employed full-time at hospitals and only worked at the RHO's clinics one or two half days a week, which meant that I sometimes needed to wait days before they could find time to speak with me again and I could get answers to the specific questions I needed to ask. However, Fatima and Kaoutar were much more accessible to me, and our interviews usually took place over lunch or after all the patients were checked in to see the doctor. More structured interviews that I recorded were conducted with staff at the main office of the RHO, at the Ministry of Health, and at various development organizations, including the United Nations Development Program (UNDP), the UN Population Fund (UNFPA), the United States Agency for International Development (USAID), and the United Nations Development Fund for Women (UNIFEM, now termed UN Women).

I found the waiting rooms to be fruitful places for conversations with female patients. The majority seemed to welcome my questions and inquisitions even after I told them what I was doing in Morocco. I did not push the ones who hesitated or who remained quiet when I introduced myself, but, overall, this did not occur too often. I began our conversations by asking why they had come to the clinic that day and then proceeded to ask open-ended questions about their everyday experiences of fertility and/or motherhood, childbearing and childrearing practices that they did or did not use, their ideas about what it means to be a "good" mother and woman, the ideal family and gender roles, the future of their children and the country, and the roles that their family members and spouses (if they were married) played in their reproductive decisions and practices. Here are just a few questions that I tended to pose to female patients: Why did you come to the clinic today? When have you come to the clinic before? What do you think of the services it provides? How many children do you have and/or how many children do you want to have? What does your husband think about children? Who comes with you to the clinic usually? What about the future for your children here in Morocco? What work does a mother do inside and outside the home? How can the services here be made better?

Out of these conversations sprung close relationships with eleven women that allowed me to follow them from the clinics into their homes. Over the course of my fieldwork, I worked with twenty-three women in their homes and local communities; this includes these patients' families, and four of the women were not originally patients at the clinics. I met them through other means, but they welcomed me into their homes nonetheless, and I included my observations and interviews in my data. I visited each of these homes at least two times over the course of six months, when I moved my research outside of the clinics, and some I visited more frequently over a longer period of time. I spent an entire afternoon or evening in their homes interacting with them and their female family members and friends as well as their male kin. By following a group of women, I was able to observe them in their daily lives and to speak with them a bit more openly about issues of fertility, pregnancy, marriage, and family when we were outside of the clinics and in a private setting. It was very useful having their families and friends participate in my research because it enabled me to understand the social context in which reproductive practices take place. Outside of the clinics, I also spoke to religious leaders, university students, and my colleagues who were fellow foreigners in Morocco living there for research or work. With their consent, I have included data from our conversations in this ethnography.

## KEY PARTICIPANTS

I would like to take some time to give details about my relationship with a few key participants and their lives. Fatima has worked as the director of the RHO clinic in Tarma since 2003. We first met in 2006 when I was an intern for the organization as part of my preliminary research and would make regular trips to the clinic to conduct observations. Fatima was a mother of a two-year-old boy named Ahmed. He accompanied her to the clinic on occasion with his nanny, Jasmina, and sometimes her husband. Fatima was married to a man who worked for the Moroccan military, and they lived in the local area. It would take Fatima about twenty minutes to get to the clinic for work via public transit.

Fatima worked closely with all of the OB/GYNs and doctors at the clinic, but she had a close relationship with Dr. Senah, who had delivered her son. Like many of the interns she allowed to work at the clinic to gain experience, Fatima received medical training at a technical school in Rabat. She was not a certified nurse, and, therefore, she could not draw blood or do any medical procedures. She did, however, assist the doctors whenever necessary as there was no nurse at the clinic. Fatima not only checked in patients each morning, but she ensured that the clinic had the right supplies and all of the patients' charts were complete and filed at the end of each day. She administered pregnancy tests and was responsible for family planning counseling. Fatima wore many different hats at the clinic, but this took a toll on her health. In the winter of 2009, she was ordered by her doctor to take a two-month hiatus from work due to physical and mental stress. She was tired and suffered from constant headaches and indigestion. During her time off, a substitute counselor named Hannen took over. She was a woman in her early thirties who helped out in the clinics around the Rabat region when necessary. The two sewing teachers at the clinic also stepped in and started doing some of the administrative tasks while Fatima was away. Hannen also trained in the local area like Fatima and worked at the organization's clinics for three years.

Kaoutar had worked as the director of the Zitounia clinic for a number of years. She has been with the organization since the late 1980s when the Zitounia clinic was first established. Kaoutar is originally from Marrakech, where she attended high school and college. She and her husband originally moved to Rabat for his job with the Moroccan government. They have two children together, a son who graduated from high school in 2008 and was attending a small technical school and a daughter who was twenty-six years old at the time and working for a large French-owned call center in Rabat. At the time of my research, both of their children still lived at home, which is located near Tarma. In 2012, her daughter was married and had moved out of the family's home. Even though Kaoutar traveled about thirty minutes each day to the clinic for work, and then back again, it was all worth it according to her. She enjoyed getting to know the women in Zitounia who attended the clinic. Oftentimes, when I would speak with a woman in the waiting room, Kaoutar would tell me that this woman had come to the clinic during her pregnancy or had accompanied another woman to the clinic previously. She knew nearly every repeat patient by name. She took great pride in helping women in the local area, especially because the clinic is located in a poorer neighborhood of the city. Kaoutar realized that the women who came to see the doctor did not have the resources as those who lived in her middle-class quarter.

The third director who I worked with was named Malika. She had been a longtime employee of the Ministry of Health and served as the head nurse of the public health clinic. She worked closely with Fatima in making sure that all men and women received the proper services that they needed at either the public health clinic or the RHO's clinic. The two would often make referrals to the other's facility. Malika, a tall woman in her mid-forties who wore the hijab along with her white lab coat to work every day, had a particular air about her. She was the authority at the public clinic and had very specific ideas as to how it should be run: a doorman policed the entrance, men and women waited their turns to see the doctor, women were patient to receive contraception, and doctors were to see patients quickly yet still offer them the best care possible. The public center was inundated with patients on a daily basis, much more than Malika thought it could handle, but she made do. This was demonstrated through her semi-strict ways of management, which included instructing me as to when I should come to the clinic: in the morning during SME when doctors vaccinated infants and nurses distributed contraception. I casually asked Malika who the free birth control pills were intended for, but I phrased my question in this way, "Are these pills for women, girls, married women, unmarried women? Can men get them?" (Sometimes men would come into the RHO clinics to pick up pills for their wives.) Malika responded firmly to my question, "No, these are for married women." (This was regardless of their age as some women are still married in their teenage years in Morocco.) Her tone was stern and she quickly turned her head away from me and went back to work distributing pills. It was obvious she was a bit upset that I even thought to ask such as question. The RHO, on the other hand, did not discriminate based on marital status in the clinics or in the outreach program.

## STATUS AND CLASS

Social science research in Morocco has shown that socioeconomic status has an impact on women's health and the care they receive (Batnitzky 2008; Boutayeb 2006). Poorer women often fare worse than wealthier women because they cannot afford to see a doctor. This is not new in the realm of global health and is common throughout the world, but I build on the work by anthropologists Vinh-Kim Nguyen and Karine Peschard (2003) to demonstrate that other social and cultural factors can produce inequalities in reproductive healthcare. It is not always just about financial resources. I believe that it is important to situate my participants in terms of social class particularly because I trace how individual practices link to larger national and international movements in development and healthcare; class can certainly impact how these connections take shape.

The large majority of the female patients from the clinics were of the working class. They were poorer urban women who ranked near the bottom of the socioeconomic scale in Morocco. They did not live in extreme poverty, such as those living in *bidonvilles* around Rabat, but they also did not have the financial resources of the wealthier classes. For example, one woman I worked with named Layla lived in a small one-bedroom apartment with her husband and her five children in Rabat. Another woman, Suad, lived in a two-story, two-bedroom apartment near Tarma with her parents, older sister, and two younger brothers. One woman I spoke with as she waited with her sister to see the doctor, Amina, said to me, "We do not have a lot, but we're okay." Not having great wealth meant these women sometimes struggled to buy goods and household items needed every day and to afford necessary health services. It also meant they could not send their children to more expensive Moroccan private schools or to international academies in Rabat run by Americans or the French. These constraints not only impacted our interactions and our conversations, but they also subsequently informed my analysis of the data I collected.

The Moroccan state has been a guardian of citizens' social mobility because it functions as a regulator and as an employer. This has sparked debate among political figures and the public about the role of the state in everyday life. Shana Cohen writes, "Individuals could 'move up' (*ytil'/ monter*) through education and a post in either the colonial or Moroccan national administration at the same time that the state, Morocco as a nation, came into being and embarked on a course of economic and social development" (2004, 36). She argues in Morocco there has been a rise of a "global middle class" partly due to market liberalization. This class challenges the nation-state. "Middle class" in Morocco does not particularly refer to a standard of living, Cohen suggests, but rather a guarantee of all life's necessities. I choose to use the term "working class" in response to this formulation because the majority of my female participants were not able to afford all of life's necessities, which Cohen describes. They constantly negotiated their economic and social circumstances within their reproductive decision making and practices.

On the other hand, the clinical staff, doctors, executive staff members at the RHO, government officials, and staff at the development agencies could be considered middle and even upper class. I am fully aware of this discrepancy between my participants and attempt to incorporate it into my ethnographic material and my analysis. However, rather than re-create feminist tropes from the mid twentieth century in which women from the developed world or the elite classes try to "save" Third-World and poor women (Jayawardena 1986; Spivak 1988), I take these class intersections as moments to examine the varied ideas of femininity and motherhood that exist in Morocco; converging and diverging discourses about religion, health, and modernity; and reproductive practices in daily life that may be similar or different between groups and individuals.

## CONCEPTUALIZING A STUDY OF REPRODUCTION THROUGH FEMINIST MEDICAL ANTHROPOLOGY

The approach that I take in this ethnography to reproductive practices and development policies is analytical yet generous. I argue the individualization and the privatization of the self that are promoted through recent development policies in Morocco have produced various interpretations of childbearing and childrearing practices among women. My female participants appropriated these practices in ways that unsuspectingly circumscribe them as being Moroccan citizens through their reproductive bodies instead of their productive labor. Policies and laws concerning women's rights and bodies in the country have constructed women, in general, as citizens in ways other than being a mother; however, medical practices and advice in the clinic and public discussions of citizenship have counteracted this process. I do agree that numerous Moroccan women want to become mothers, as women do in other parts of the world, and some women do not or cannot, but my focus is on: What are the characteristics and behaviors of modern reproductive subjects and citizens in Morocco, and how do these differ between individuals? How can we analyze these in the context of transnational discourses of reproduction, health, and development? What do people mean when they talk about the future of the Morocco and the roles that childbearing and childrearing play in it? How do women appropriate the childbearing and childrearing practices promoted in the clinics and by the state?

In answering these questions, I draw heavily on scholarship in medical anthropology in order to take a critical approach to reproduction. In commemorating the fiftieth anniversary of the field, Marcia Inhorn writes that one objective of medical anthropologists has been to "look at . . . the structural violence triggered by processes of globalization, neoliberalism, and global capitalism. In the midst of these macrostructural forces, medical anthropologists have examined the social construction of illness categories, the individual illness narratives used to articulate these, and the social and political hierarchies such categories may produce or maintain" (2010, 264). Medical anthropology and feminist theory have long worked in tandem (Bray 2007; Cameron 2010; Lock and Kaufert 1998). The topic of reproduction (i.e., fertility and infertility, contraception, pregnancy, medical technologies, etc.) has been a site at which these two fields have come together quite frequently (Davis 2009; Layne 2003; Markens 2007). Janelle Taylor states that feminist ethnographers of reproduction have in fact accomplished what anthropologists have long tried to show: "that to study ordinary people in their everyday lives is, indeed, to address 'big ideas.' As they go about the social work of reproducing new generations and struggling to build and maintain healthy lives, families, and communities, women also engage in the imagining and producing culture and social relations" (2004, 130). "Big ideas" is central to my analysis in this ethnography. In building on work in medical anthropology, I situate my female participants' reproductive practices in national discourses of development and global discourses of reproductive health and fertility. For my purposes, I bring together approaches and theory from medical anthropology and feminist studies to provide a framework in order to question meanings of citizenship, definitions of femininity, constructions of gender, and the most recent development agenda in Morocco.

Throughout this ethnography, I engage with medical anthropologists who locate reproduction at the center of their analyses in order to open up broader questions about what Taylor calls "big ideas." Ginsburg and Rapp suggest that by using reproduction as an entry point for study, scholars can see how "cultures are produced (or contested) as people imagine an enable the creation of the next generation, most directly through the nurturance of children" (1995, 1–2). Over the course of my fieldwork, I learned that my Moroccan female participants did not talk about development in terms of their own lives, but rather discussed how the reproductive practices they employed today could be used to improve the lives of their children. Given this, the use and nonuse of such practices showed how they imagined the future generation and produced culture. Shifting focus from reproduction within a specific culture or group to reproduction across cultures and groups allows for a better understanding of how the global and the local intersect, or perhaps these are not as clear-cut categories as once thought. This ethnography is built on three levels: the national/international, the institutional, and the individual. They are in constant conversation with each other throughout this text. "Stratified reproduction" is very useful to think with here because it allows me to delineate which bodies come to count and which do not when the local, global, national, and individual levels intersect with one another in the areas of Rabat in which I worked. This concept, discussed by Shellee Colen (1995), refers to the hierarchy of birth, reproductive health services, and childrearing that encourages some women to become mothers while discouraging others. I challenge the theorization of reproduction as a universal aspect of womanhood (cf. Davis-Floyd and Sargent 1997; Inhorn 1994) and build on work that has taken issue with this argument and offered alternative ways of thinking about gender and the female body (Berend 2010; Kahn 2000; Morell 1994). In doing so, I open up a space to theorize childbearing and childrearing practices as outside of biological determinants and instead within a realm composed of political moves and social constructions.

I draw on work in medical anthropology and feminist studies that address the relationship between medical discourses and gender, on the one hand, and the ways that culture and society impact medical practices, on the other. My analysis is informed by a call by Donna Haraway (1988) for an examination of knowledge that is both "situated" and embodied and that takes into serious consideration the multiple perspectives of officials, providers, and citizens at once. I draw inspiration from scholarship in medical anthropology that complicates inequality and reframes health disparities (Cohen 1999; Farmer 2004; Gravlee 2009; Petryna 2005). Moreover, I use this scholarship to challenge the common assumption found in much public health literature that poverty is the primary hindrance to accessing regular healthcare in Morocco. Rapp notes, "Feminist attention to embodied inequalities quickly focused on reproduction as a site of investigation and intervention" (2001, 466). Nguyen and Peschard argue, "A distinction has been made between social relations, where the violence of inequality is most often expressed in ritualized form, leaving visible traces on the body, and those where the violence of inequality is transcribed into the body as biological difference and expressed as 'risk' to be managed through techniques of government" (2003, 448). They offer an alternative for understanding inequality that is outside of economic status. My female participants, although working class, faced numerous cultural and social constraints in their quest for reproductive health services. I argue that these constraints are deeply engrained in how they have come to think of themselves as Moroccan citizens, as women, and as mothers. Some women could not receive care because only a male doctor was on staff that day, whereas others refused the IUD because of their husbands' dismay with the device; I will go into detail about these occurrences later in the text.

Family planning, pregnancy, reproductive technologies, infertility, and motherhood are recurrent topics in medical anthropology (Adams 1994; Boddy 1989; Fleuriet 2009; Fordyce 2012; Hughes 2011). However, there is much less work that concentrates on the aggregate level. Whereas I do focus on the individual practices of reproduction and motherhood, I do so in order to show how Moroccan women are being configured as modern subjects within the population. One of my research questions was: What are the reproductive subjects that are being produced through human development? Work that has examined the population has often engaged with biopower, a concept put forth most notably by Michel Foucault (1990). Foucault shows that biopower takes human beings as its objects of study and intervention and characterizes them as members of the population. He writes, "The disciplines of the body and the regulations of the population constituted the two poles around which the organization of power over life was deployed" (1990, 139). The well-being of the population became a major objective for the government, Foucault suggests, as did the management of the population as a whole (Ali 2002; Chatterjee and Riley 2001; Greenhalgh 2003; Krause 2005; Langford 2009). In their comprehensive study of China's population program and one-child policy, Susan Greenhalgh and Edwin Winckler (2005) propose three subjects are produced through the policy and governmental practices: the reproductive woman, the good mother, and the quality child. In Morocco, numerous women's magazine articles that have appeared in recent years have explicitly discussed proper reproductive and mothering practices, which are to be utilized in order to raise healthy children who will be able to enhance society in the future. Examples include those from the section *Votre Enfant* (Your Child) in the popular magazine *Femmes du Maroc*.

One parallel between Morocco and the China case is that there was not a single one-child policy in China (Greenhalgh 2008), and in Morocco there has not been one single all-encompassing policy concerning reproduction or development, but rather at times conflicting initiatives and discourses that must be pieced together. Still, I contend the "messiness" of this process facilitates the production of new subjects and ways of being in the population. I detail the new subjects being produced—citizens, women, and mothers—and highlight the multiplicities that exist within each. Although an in-depth study of the ways that strict government policies about contraception and abortion bled into women's everyday lives in Romania, Gail Kligman's (1998) very powerful book *The Politics of Duplicity: Controlling Reproduction in Ceausescu's Romania* also focuses on the repressive aspects of biopower and frames such a regime as disciplining and negative. Kligman conveys biopower as strictly a repressive force in society sometimes abused by officials, but I complicate this theorization and build on work like that by Greenhalgh and Winckler (2005) to show biopower is also positive and productive. When public policy intersects with social and cultural forces, and I focus on Islam and class in Morocco, it creates new and complex bodies, selves, and ways of thinking about citizenship.

## THE HUMAN BODY

During the course of her lifetime, a woman's body goes through many physical changes. A woman who attends health clinics or accepts certain childbearing practices may change the way her body appears or feels in ways that coincide with discourses that are culturally and historically specific.

Helen Gremillion poses that bodies are "constructed: they are thoroughly embedded in culturally normalized, gendered ideals" (2003, 33). In my study, such ideals surround womanhood, femininity, fertility, the family, and reproduction. Gremillion (2003) argues though that when we theorize the body in this way, very difficult questions come about: What are the material stakes involved? How do we analyze the body without relying on biological functions? How can we talk about the physical risks involved in reproduction while situating them in broader discourses? These questions are not specific to just studies of reproduction; they reiterate feminist scholars' overall concern for the need to speak to "big ideas" of society through the lens of women's bodies.

I consider the lived experiences and material realities of my female participants and the clinical staff carefully (Zhan 2005) given that childbearing and childrearing practices cannot be explained adequately through biomedical discourses alone. They can only be understood as such discourses intersect with cultural, political, and historical ones and individuals' everyday circumstances. How can I understand a woman's desire to use contraception because she believes it is a marker of piety? How can I analyze the Moroccan government's intention to lower the TFR through human development? In trying to address these questions, it is dangerous to lose sight of the physical human body. Literature in Science and Technology Studies in particular has grappled with this conundrum as it surveys topics such as virtual worlds, new medical technologies, and novel means of communication (Boellstorff 2008; Haring 2003; Lock et al. 2000; Reed 2005). Elly Teman (2010), in her study of surrogacy and in vitro fertilization (IVF) in Israel, problematizes this conflict in her attempt to explain the experiences of local surrogate mothers within a global culture of surrogacy. Teman writes, "Examining how surrogates and intended mothers negotiate maternity, kin relations, bodies, and boundaries in a context where these stakes are so high amplifies what we might find among surrogacy participants in other cultural contexts. This local version of a global set of surrogacy practices has important implications for the human experience of surrogacy in general" (2010, 6). I draw on this work to suggest it is by looking at individual childbearing and childrearing practices that we can understand how the reproductive body is entangled within and a product of public policy and various societal discourses.

We are simultaneously human beings and social beings (Scheper-Hughes and Lock 1987). Nancy Krieger argues that once we recognize this fact, then "embodiment" puts forth three claims: bodies are able to tell us stories that are not separate from our "conditions of existence," bodies tell stories that "match people's stated accounts," and bodies tell stories that "people cannot or will not tell" (2005, 350). Many scholars, myself included, have concern with constructionist accounts of the body, but it is not so much that they exclude the physical body or everyday experiences, but that the body—constructed or not—always carries with it a specific and marked meaning (Lugo and Maurer 2000; Ortner 1974; Zhan 2005). Even though I agree with constructionist approaches that challenge the naturalness of the body, I believe that they gloss over what we physically experience as humans (Rosaldo 1974). "Deconstructing" the body is an important analytical step; however, it "does not allow for a consideration of the social and cultural practices that render the body a seemingly natural object . . . some constructionists fall short on their own terms by reinscribing the body as an acultural 'thing'" (Gremillion 2003, 35). Engaging with work in medical anthropology that focuses on what "embodiment" means (Cooper et al. 2003; Garcia 2008; Volk 2009; Zhan 2009) has allowed me to question reproductive practices and bodies not just as products, but rather as a mixture of "naturalness" and dominant cultural discourses that make the body seem like a "natural thing." This is an imperative part of my project given that women in Morocco tend to be constructed as citizens through their reproductive bodies—their abilities to control and enhance the country's population.

The idea of the human body as a cultural product is critical to studies of medicine, and at the same time, it is just as important to recognize that culture impacts the treatment and diagnoses of bodies (Montoya 2007). This ethnography illustrates how state policies and programs, medical providers, and development agencies actively produce specific kinds of bodies that fit within the model of the modern citizen in Morocco. The processes behind adopting particular modern reproductive practices vary from group to group. Many of the women I worked with envisioned similar goals as the government and development agencies when it came to the future of Morocco, but they phrased them in ways that made sense to their own daily lives. Moreover, I show that the reproductive body is produced through cultural and medical processes. This is where it is important that I do not lose sight of daily reproductive practices because I am suggesting that they already existed but were not specifically defined or talked about in terms of an individualized and privatized self until the launch of the INDH. I propose that the practices promoted in the medical facilities where I conducted research by staff and by development programs (both medical and nonmedical in nature) create particular understandings of citizenship that come from and are embedded within changing global discourses of development and reproduction.

Donna Haraway writes, "These claims are on people's lives. I am arguing for the view from a body; always complex, contradictory, structuring, and structured body, versus the view from above, from nowhere, from simplicity" (1988, 589). On many different occasions, some of my participants would talk about contraception and reproductive healthcare in ways that situated Morocco in between Europe, the United States, Africa, and the MENA. They discussed such practices as drawing them closer to one region while simultaneously distancing them from another, but this was not a linear movement. They created ways of belonging for themselves that were always in motion between different regions and the dominant discourses they associated with each. How can I understand this? How can I explore the historical past of European colonialism, the country's current political and economic relationships, and Moroccans' connection to Islam using contraception? Why do some Moroccans talk about childbearing and childrearing practices in this way? Bringing together constructionist accounts with a "view from the body" proposed by Haraway provides me with the analytic tools to explore lived experiences of reproduction, and at the same time, locate these experiences and the body at a particular historical and cultural place (Gremillion 2003; Zhan 2009). Moroccans and their bodies have always been located within this space where various regions and cultures clash or converge. This approach also allows me to historicize my arguments without reifying the past and to critically analyze how women are articulating and repackaging "older" concerns in new ways that fit their individual contexts.

Women's bodies have long been considered by feminist scholars to be central to the collective's identity, and in this ethnography, I demonstrate how women's reproductive practices and the control (either by the self or through intervention) of their reproductive bodies has come in part to define Moroccan modernity. One may argue that their bodies embody the nation. Yuval-Davis, in her book *Gender and Nation*, argues that women are the "symbolic border guards" (1997, 61) of the nation; their bodies allow individuals to enter or to be denied acceptance. This is a powerful conception of the body. The female body here cannot be described as separate from the construction of the nation, especially since, as Yuval-Davis argues, people are born into the collective. Throughout this text, I engage with the idea that women's bodies are of particular importance to the defining of Morocco (and I suggest that a second project could think through how ideas of masculinity enter in this process). Suad Joseph (1999) links notions of womanhood to constructions of citizenship in Lebanon. She argues that women are able to cross boundaries and position themselves in several communities at once, thus creating spaces for resistance to a male and elite nationalism. I do not disagree that the female body is a site of nation building, but I propose that it is necessary to destabilize the "naturalization" of nation and woman in modernity and instead consider how the very processes of gendering of the body and the citizen play into the construction of the nation.

## INDIVIDUAL CHOICE

Individual choice over one's body is a highly complicated and contested matter with no clear-cut answers. For example, Angela Garcia demonstrates that heroin use and overdose among individuals living in New Mexico is not just a matter of choosing whether or not to engage in such a behavior; it is deeply rooted in the region's economic and social histories. Even though "the motivating factor behind drug recovery is invariably understood in terms of personal choice or will" (2008, 727), Garcia argues that in order to treat heroin use successfully, this past must be put into conversation with the present to understand what this "choice or will" means. Similarly, Carole Browner (2001) masterfully argues that although "social structures" may have a direct impact on women's reproductive decisions and practices, it would be unproductive to assume that they are the only factors. Drawing on ethnographic research from the United States, Colombia, and Mexico, Browner suggests that these structures are interpreted and become meaningful through "cultural processes" about gender and women. Both these "cultural processes" and "structural factors" need to be taken into account when studying women's reproductive choices.

The notion of women's choice in Morocco has been framed in the literature primarily in terms of how women work to resist and subvert patriarchal structures of power. Rachel Newcomb, in her book *Women of Fes: Ambiguities of Urban Life in Morocco*, writes, "The outliers succeed when they are able to translate their actions into idioms comprehensible to others who would be quick to reject innovations perceived as completely foreign to Moroccan culture. In other words, working within the existing structures of power to gain acceptance for something new was often absolutely necessary" (2008, 5). Similarly, Loubna Skalli (2001) argues economic, social, cultural, and legal structures of Morocco have worked against women, thus forcing a relatively large portion of the female population into poverty. Skalli points out the *Plan d'Action pour l'Intégration des Femmes au Développement* (Plan of Action for Integrating Women in Development) "does not target poverty in its narrowest meaning of the term; rather, it seeks to adopt a holistic approach to many ills from which women suffer at the economic, legal, and socio-cultural levels" (2001, 86). The objective is to release working-class and poverty-stricken women from structural constraints in order to allow them to make a wider range of choices for themselves. Bernhard Venema and Jogien Bakker (2004) argue the common assumption that Muslim women inhabit a male-dominant society and that control over women's sexual practices and bodies enhance men's status has come to be highly relevant in Morocco due to the process of Islamization. This combined with social conditions, including being of a lower socio-economic class, leads women with few choices and alternatives in reality. Venema and Bakker explore the option of prostitution in their article, but make the argument that the conditions of possibility through which such a profession exists and thrives are rampant in Morocco.

As these authors demonstrate in their work on Morocco, the idea of individual choice, although argued to be a neoliberal and modern concept (Burchell 1996; Rose and Miller 2008), is more complicated than having or not having choice. Cultural forces, political economy, and historical constructions of gender must be taken into account when discussing women's choices over their bodies. Although I find the work by the authors mentioned in the preceding extremely valuable, I problematize the notion that women in Morocco are working to just resist patriarchal power structures by foregrounding familial struggles and social prescriptions that complicate their decisions, or even their abilities to decide. Work on reproductive decision making has taken up this point, for example, Carolyn Sargent's (2006) study of Malian migrants in Paris. The family's desire to have children is in contrast to the French medical system's encouragement to limit their number of children. This comparison makes women's decisions anything but ordinary and forces them to adopt new interpretations of Islam in order to quell these conflicts. A seminal work on this topic is the book *Taking Chances: Abortion and the Decision Not to Contracept* by Kristin Luker (1991). Luker demonstrates how the abortion debate in the United States, particularly in California, became more about the activities of women and their "moral claim to end their pregnancies." Some cases of abortion are tolerated whereas others are not depending upon the circumstances surrounding the pregnancy (such as pregnancies that resulted from incest or rape). Luker writes, "Put another way, a woman who does not 'take care of herself' by using contraception is often seen as having compromised her claim to an abortion" (1991, ix). Luker includes detailed flowcharts concerning women's decision-making processes in her text. She argues the notion of choice is "messy" and involved. Whereas some debates highlight this point, others erase it completely.

In this ethnography, I build on the work of Luker in that I agree choice is very complicated and difficult to define; however, my goal here is not to particularly highlight the debates about reproductive practices, including abortion, but to destabilize the idea in political and scholarly discourses that neoliberal reforms and constructions of the individualized self actually produce a wider range of choices for individuals about their bodies. When the transition occurs from the welfare state to neoliberal forms of governance, the government is to take a step back from people's everyday lives, thus producing new subjectivities (Comaroff and Comaroff 2001; Kanna 2010; Sawyer 2004; Sharma 2006). My ethnography demonstrates that in the context of working-class Moroccan women's lives, it is not about choosing or not choosing to do the "right thing," but there are both cultural and structural barriers that these women must tackle in the process of making the "right" decisions that will ultimately lead to the improvement of their well-being, that of their family, and that of Morocco. Later in the text, I argue that rhetoric of responsibility and self-governance actually produces further fear and anxiety among my female participants concerning their reproductive practices and mothering due to the conflicting social, cultural, religious, and economic discourses they must navigate. This leads me to critically examine how the promise of human development to help individuals achieve their maximum potential—a stepping-stone for economic growth—is being experienced by my female participants in their daily lives.

Tropes of choice and individualism have moved across national and transnational neoliberal discourses of rights, development, politics, and economics. I am not arguing that neoliberalism allows for individuals to do as they please; on the contrary, neoliberal logic creates alternative ways to discipline bodies by using the community, civil society, the family, and the self. Anthropological studies that take up the question of neoliberalism often draw upon the concept of "governmentality" as delineated by Foucault (1991), to describe how subjects are regulated and a logic of self-governance is produced. In her study of work and family life in Poland, Marysia Galbraith (2008) argues neoliberal values of individualism and responsibility are in conflict with the cultural significance of children and the family. This contradiction, coupled with the lack of social support for Poles, produces a "climate of insecurity" that has led to the country's declining birthrate. Galbraith writes, "The challenges Polish women face fulfilling roles as both parents and workers reflect a society-level failure to reconcile prenatal values that shape social policy with neoliberal capitalist ideology" (2008, 17). In this ethnography, my questions are: How does this neoliberal rhetoric of the self as an individual intersect with the "messiness" of women's choices concerning their reproductive practices? What type of self evolves out of this intersection? How does this impact women's everyday practices and decisions concerning childbearing and childrearing? What does it mean for them? What about the women's husbands or families, or what about their own desire to have more children? These types of questions are missing from the neoliberal discourses of development and health in Morocco.

## NEOLIBERALISM AND ISLAM

Although the scholarship on neoliberalism is vast (Elyachar 2005; Ferguson 2006; Harvey 2007; Ong 2006), there is actually very little work on the intersection of religious beliefs and practices with neoliberal transformations. Scholars have studied religious revival and resurgence (Buckser 1996; Fernando 2010; Hirschkind 2006) and a great deal of work has focused on globalization and transnational shifts in modes of governance (Appadurai 1996; Ong 1999), but relatively few scholars have put religion, neoliberalism, and globalization in the same framework.

Stephen Collier and Aihwa Ong (2005), in their edited volume *Global Assemblages: Technology, Politics, and Ethics as Anthropological Problems*, demonstrate that neoliberalism operates according to the rationality of a certain market type. Through the collection of essays, they show that the shape of neoliberalism, and its significance for individuals and collectives, can only be understood as it enters into "assemblages" with other elements in society. Ong and Collier's suggestion is seductive because it forces us to study neoliberalism in its different variations and within particular contexts, but religion was not a main focus of the chapters even though I believe it is an important factor in how neoliberalism is defined, perceived, and interpreted. Whereas I find the concept of the "assemblage" to be useful in order to not do the "God-trick" and define neoliberalism from above, at the same time, I also believe the concept assumes it is predefined and only transforms as it intersects with other forces in society. This ethnography illustrates that neoliberalism is not just morphed; its definition and salience are produced within these entanglements. My main contribution here to the study of neoliberalism is to think through a conception of neoliberal Islam or Islamic neoliberalism within the Moroccan context, a place nearly absent from the literature on neoliberalism to begin with.

I build on the existing scholarship on neoliberalism in order to theorize the importance of civil society and the individual self in the production of modern citizens in Morocco—who are defined by the state and institutions involved in development as self-regulating and self-governing. Dr. Binjal, one of the founders of the RHO, believes the involvement of civil society and IOs in reproductive health has been essential for Morocco to lower the TFR and the population growth rate; however, he also feels the government has become dependent on such aid in order to accomplish its agenda. Nikolas Rose (1999), in his work on neoliberalism in the West, examines the paradox of neoliberalism that Dr. Binjal describes. Rose argues the rationale behind the reconfiguration of the state was ultimately economic. The state was taking on projects that could be better handled by the private sector or civil society, and, in the case of Morocco, this was reproductive health and family planning. Rose states, "To govern better, the state must govern less; to optimize the economy, one must govern through the entrepreneurship of autonomous actors—individuals and families, firms and corporations" (1999, 139). The step back taken by the state in Morocco in terms of reproductive health was intended to help create an atmosphere that was, and continues to be, conducive to individuals' acceptance of reproductive health services, medical technologies, and family planning on their own terms.

In this process, Moroccans will become modern and responsible citizens who govern their reproductive behaviors and make decisions that will not only improve their lives, but also will enhance the nation and its future. Aradhana Sharma, in her work on women's empowerment in India, notes the presence of "quasi- and nonstate actors in India and their conjoining with state-sponsored grassroots empowerment initiatives reflect, in certain respects global neoliberal trends that seek to 'autonomize' entities of government from state institution by spreading techniques of self-government throughout social space" (2006, 64). What Sharma demonstrates in her work is that through partial "degovernmentalization" (Barry et al. 1996) neoliberalism creates citizen-subjects who are "active" (Rose 1999) in making choices to further their own interests, but this is done unknowingly in the name of the larger collective. This point is critical to my larger project here.

Neoliberalism has been taken up in many different ways: an ideology, a set of economic practices, and a rationality of government (Mitchell 2002; Rofel 2007; Speed 2005). Some scholarship on the topic has examined neoliberalism in relation to Marxist traditions (Harvey 2007; Peterson 2001), and other work has discussed the rise of neoliberalism within the context of Foucault's governmentality (Lakoff 2005; Rabinow 1995). But the literature I draw upon most in formulating this ethnography is that which does not address neoliberalism per se, but focuses on the practices that follow such logic (Ellison 2009; Kanna 2010; Maurer 2005; Sunder-Rajan 2006). I do not theorize neoliberalism as abstract. Instead I elucidate the very practices that are constitutive of it. I start by closely examining the childbearing and childrearing practices promoted and discussed by the government, development organizations, medical providers, community members, outreach workers, and the media, which opens up a space for me to analyze what neoliberalism and "neoliberal citizens" mean within the context of Morocco. Doing so forces me to not predefine neoliberalism, but rather to concentrate on the intersection of various practices and multiple discourses in order to find its significance.

In beginning from the premise that neoliberalism can be understood only through practice, I argue that in Morocco, neoliberal transformations and Islamic ideals must be kept within the same frame, and, by doing so, we see these are not two contradictory discourses. Anthropologists have successfully illustrated that Islamic beliefs and practices can impact people's decisions regarding the use of "new" reproductive practices and technologies (Inhorn 2004; Johnson-Hanks 2006b), but I argue Islam not only informs reproductive behaviors, but individuals' interpretations of Islam are just as equally influenced by the introduction and acceptance of particular childbearing and childrearing practices. I delineate one way of looking at what might be termed Islamic neoliberalism or neoliberal Islam. Daromir Rudnyckyj (2009), in his work on what he calls "spiritual economies" in Indonesia, contributes to the development of this concept. Rudnyckyj states, "spiritual economies refer to projects that seek to simultaneously transform workers into more religious subjects and more productive economic subjects" (2009, 106). Building on this conceptualization by Rudnyckyj, I analyze childbearing and childrearing practices (gynecological exams, contraception, ultrasounds, and counseling sessions) to demonstrate that the pious subject and the neoliberal self-governing subject are one and the same for many of my female participants, which leads me to argue that these women are seeking out alternative ways and meanings of being responsible that do not particularly stem from the development rhetoric or policies. I suggest "new" reproductive technologies and practices are actually already pious in nature for many Moroccan women precisely because they follow a neoliberal logic. This logic captures and is captured by Islamic beliefs and practices that foreground the importance of living a full and quality life.

For instance, a young female university student who was originally from Saudi Arabia, but had moved to Morocco to attend college, stated, "When I first came here and saw condoms being passed out at the student center I didn't know what to think. Aren't they going to make people have sex? That is forbidden by Islam except if they are married. But then, after a while, I realized that using a condom is actually the right thing to do and we can still be Muslims. Islam wants you to do good." This college student was concerned that condoms would actually make people have sexual relations outside of marriage, which would violate Islam. However, with time, she figured out that using a condom is not against Islam because it encourages doing "good." Likewise, at the one clinic of the RHO in Rabat, a married woman named Eisha who was in her early thirties told me while she was waiting for the counselor, "I am Muslim, but I use the pill." I asked if this was proper or "good" (*mzyan*). She responded with, "Islam wants the best. If you read the Qur'an you will see. Have you read the Qur'an?" Eisha's statement exemplifies the production of a new discourse surrounding reproduction that brings together neoliberal logic of self-regulation with the ideals of Islam concerning human life and the body. It is through my examination of how Eisha discusses the pill and the university student talks about condoms—the practices—that I can argue neoliberalism and Islam are two intersecting discourses in many Moroccan women's lives (both of the upper and working classes). This intersection produces new types of citizens who embody various representations of modernity.

## THE BOOK'S ORGANIZATION

One of my main objectives in this work is to describe and interpret daily practices in the health clinics and women's homes and the experiences that women, medical providers, state officials, and development workers discussed in interviews and that I observed in action. The participants in this ethnography are part of a larger story and discourses about reproductive health, development, gender, and citizenship. This story includes policy making and politics at the national and transnational levels; rapidly changing cultural values in the face of globalization; and new meanings of feminine citizenship that are produced through the entanglement of development programs and medical, religious, economic, and social discourses.

Chapter 1 examines the relationship between reproduction and development policies in Morocco. It also outlines a historical account of gender and development in Morocco. Beginning with the country's focus on economic development in the building of a modern nation-state in 1956, it analyzes the Moroccan state's development and implementation of various development programs over the past fifty years and demonstrates that women's reproductive bodies have been consistently at the center even though the government acknowledges they have often been "forgotten" or on the periphery in modernization. I show that reproduction has always been a critical element to development, whether the policies focus on economic or social development as there was a shift from the former to the latter come the 1990s with the new regime under King Mohammed VI, who succeeded his father, King Hassan II. I put reproductive politics and development policies side by side in this chapter to illustrate that one did not come before the other, but they developed in tandem. I show there is actually a paradox occurring in Morocco: the bigger push towards modernization, building better infrastructure, and creating more jobs—what is thought to allow people greater choices and more opportunities to succeed—actually brings about stricter controls over women's reproductive bodies.

Chapter 2 builds on the interplay of reproductive politics and development policies examined in Chapter 1, and through an examination primarily of popular culture, schoolbooks, and literacy textbooks examines the ways in which neoliberal ideas of development are pragmatically forming modern reproductive citizens. Drawing on feminist analyses and critiques of nationalism, critical studies of reproduction, and analyses of the relationship between Islam and modernity, this chapter examines how the notion of the modern citizen is being framed in terms of gender, reproduction, and faith. It focuses on ideals of reproduction and notions of proper womanhood and motherhood as depicted by images and texts. A key theme to these texts' images is the importance of autonomy and personal choice. In several of them, practices and beliefs that are associated with Islam are shown as being in opposition to using a form of contraception, and therefore a challenge to the creation of the modern Moroccan citizen.

Chapter 3 will provide an overview of the reproductive health clinics and outreach programs, giving the reader a sense of how patients come under the medical and governmental gaze. How does a policy become embodied? How is the development rhetoric carried out in everyday practice on behalf of the medical providers and patients? What sights and sounds contribute to the creation of the modern reproductive subject and modern citizen in Morocco? This chapter is intended to introduce the audience to the spaces of intervention in which I conducted fieldwork and the interventionist reproductive practices that were deployed in them, such as charting, triage, counseling sessions, the examinations by doctors, and dispensing of contraception. The next three chapters will build upon this one in that they will show how women actually appropriate these practices of intervention to create new identities, understandings of Islam, and ideas of womanhood and motherhood in ways unintended by the Moroccan government, NGOs, and national and international development agencies, but that are nonetheless still within the development rubric of responsibility and active participation.

Whereas Part I of my ethnography (Chapters 1 to 3) takes a broader overview of the ways Morocco is trying to create modern reproductive subjects and citizens, Part II looks at how this process is being carried out in the everyday lives of working-class women in Rabat. Drawing on observations of the medical encounter between medical providers and female patients who sought reproductive healthcare and on interviews with both providers and patients, Chapter 4 illustrates the ways that popular understandings of Islam converge with the economic conditions of working-class Moroccan women in their decisions to accept modern methods of family planning, most notably the birth control pill (the most popular method in the country). Living a quality life and being able to provide such a life to your children are tenets in both the new social development policy in Morocco and in Islam. Beginning with Karl Marx, theorists have suggested that economic circumstances and religious beliefs are hierarchical. When it comes to making decisions about healthcare, financial matters trump religion. However, I show that these two domains are actually held in the same frame by working-class female patients at the clinics as well as some healthcare providers. Poorer Moroccan women who attended the clinics adopt the neoliberal ideals of responsibility and exhibiting self-control when it comes to family building, meaning that they will not have more children than they can provide for adequately. My ethnographic research shows that they interpret these beliefs through religious discourses and will couch their reasons for using contraception within their understandings of Islamic tenets surrounding fertility and motherhood.

Chapter 5 focuses on women's reactions to their positive or negative pregnancy tests in the health clinics. Two of the clinics where I conducted fieldwork performed rapid pregnancy tests. Feminist scholars who have studied the meaning of children for women in Morocco note that children often are equated with women's roles in the family and their status in society. I do not dispute this observation, but, through careful observations of women's reactions to their test results, this chapter suggests that the meanings of womanhood and motherhood have changed with the coming of new development policies that focus on transforming the lives of citizens instead of economic growth. The vast majority of women were thrilled to discover they were not pregnant if they had two or more children; they were visibly upset when they heard they were expecting for the third, fourth, or fifth time. Whereas women were happy to know they were not going to be mothers again or mothers at a young age, what I point to in this chapter is that they frequently called on God, often noting that God understands they cannot physically or financially bear another mouth to feed and therefore that is why they are not pregnant. This was often in reference to Islam's stress on the fact that God does not want to burden anyone or to give them hardships (found in the Qur'an); however, the Moroccan government as well as medical providers advocate that citizens need to make the right decisions about their bodies and children.

Using ethnographic data and popular culture, Chapter 6 asks: How do Moroccan women envision the future of the country? What are the characteristics of the next generation of modern citizens in their eyes? It takes the waiting room in the health clinics as a space where definitions of motherhood are reconfigured to fit within the rapid modernization that the country is experiencing because this is where women can talk freely and engage in friendly debates about childrearing and their everyday lives. I examine these novel ideas of modern motherhood that come out of these conversations, and then I trace how these definitions are put into practice as I recount my observations of women and their families in their homes and local communities. I show that to be modern and successful in the future, children must be taught how to live a more prosperous and economically viable life, but they must also be taught how to be moral, how to further their religious knowledge, and how to have "good hearts." Religious knowledge and material wealth are not separate from one another for the women I observed and interviewed, but they go hand in hand in raising the next generation. I show childrearing is just one more way that women have appropriated the neoliberal rhetoric of development to create new meanings of what good motherhood means and new definitions of the modern child.

Drawing from the Moroccan experience, the conclusion theorizes the ways in which states use the reproductive body as a means of creating "ideal" and modern citizens through the inculcation of neoliberal values and ideas. The conclusion illustrates that Moroccan women feel an uncertainty when it comes to the future in regards to their bodies and the bodies of their children because of the additional social, political, and economic pressures put on them to raise the future generations. They need to be responsible and to self-regulate their fertility in order to be "good" mothers and citizens, but sometimes this is difficult given their financial resources and social situations. Rather than relying on sociobiological or psychological models to explain why women become mothers and why they use particular childbearing and childrearing practices, we need to examine the roles of governments, policies, development agencies, culture, and social norms in creating modern reproductive subjects.

# Part I

# 1 "Dragging" Reproduction to the Center
## Development and Reproductive Policies in Morocco

In June 2008, the cover of the international news magazine *L'Express* read "Special on Morocco: The Duel Tradition-Modernity." Five young women stand in front of the Hassan II Mosque in Casablanca, one of the largest mosques in the world after Mecca and Medina. Built between 1986 and 1993 and named for the country's king during construction, Hassan II, the mosque can hold up to twenty-five thousand worshipers at one time.[1] Three women in the foreground are dressed in skirts or jeans with sweaters, whereas the women in the background pair teal-colored hijabs with long skirts. The article "La Fracture Morale" (The Moral Divide) that accompanies this image highlights the struggle between religious revival and secularism in Morocco and states that the two sides are trying to find a balance in a peaceful manner.[2] The magazine cover and article highlight that religion is just one of the many lines along which public debates emerge in Morocco. Equally as important, they emphasize that women's bodies are the means by which political and social struggles are carried out and the outcomes are gauged. I borrow a term here from Rhoda Kanaaneh (2002), who sums this up nicely in her work on Palestinian women's fertility in Israel. She describes women's bodies as "fields of contests" through which the nation along with its conflicts are inscribed.

There is an interesting paradox occurring with regards to control over women's reproductive bodies. Elizabeth Krause and Milena Marchesi (2007), in their study of population politics in Italy and its crisis of an extremely low birthrate, found that "from public critiques to personal conversations, a common organizing principle merged: the trope of oppressive Islamic regimes as the antithesis of Western modernity" (2007, 357). It is believed that "many states ruled by Sharia [seek] control over women's bodies" (Bologenetti 2004, cited in Krause and Marchesi 2007, 357). Morocco is not ruled strictly by Sharia law, but its legal system is a mix of French secular law and Sharia, which is only prevalent in the arenas of family, marriage, and divorce (Weingartner 2005). Morocco has attempted to rid itself of the image of being oppressive to women and promote itself as a liberal and modernizing Islamic nation. Part of this, I suggest, stems from the "crisis" of identity (Cohen 2004) that the country has faced since independence, as the government and

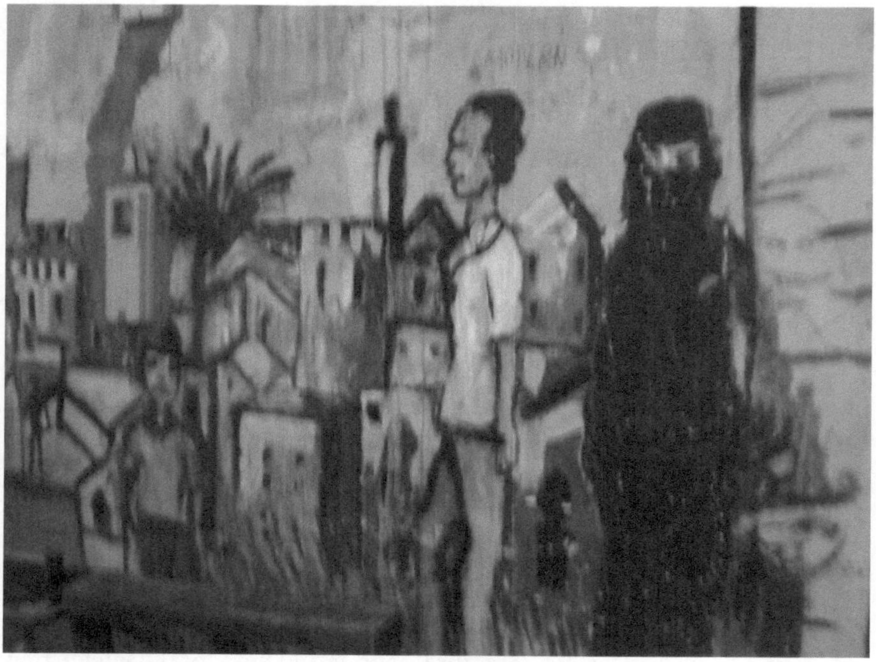

*Figure 1.1* An anonymous mural in Tangiers. (Photo by author).

citizens try to figure out what the country's role is as an interlocutor between Europe, Africa, the Middle East, and North America. In the 1990s and in 2004, as I will discuss later, Morocco reformed its personal status code, the *Moudawana*, based on Islamic Law in order to give women greater rights in marriage and divorce, and in 2007, it changed its nationality code so that mothers can also pass along citizenship to their children in addition to fathers. However, I believe that women's bodies have become central to this identity "crisis," and whereas Morocco has tried to put forth the image that it has "liberated" women through modernization and made tremendous strides in the realm of women's rights, the government, the medical community, and agencies involved in development have actually exhibited greater control over women's bodies in order for this image to be produced.

Women's bodies—and more importantly their reproductive bodies—have always been at the center of public policy and modernization efforts in Morocco. Since 1956, the year Morocco achieved independence from France, health and development policies implemented by the government have had the intention of enhancing the future of all Moroccan citizens, but such policies have covertly paid close attention to women as a way to illustrate Morocco's "modern" status to the world (Krause and Marchesi 2007). Through this, the government has incorporated women into development and constructed them as Moroccan citizens primarily through their bodily practices and their reproductive behaviors. In development, their productive labor has been made secondary to their abilities to slow population growth and decrease the TFR.

This chapter tells the story of how reproduction was "dragged" (Rapp 2001) into the heart of the Moroccan government's social and economic concerns. Reproduction lies at the center of the government's shift from economic development to social development, which was at its height in the late 1990s and early twenty-first century. This shift also in part gave rise to reproductive health programs that concentrate on creating responsible citizens instead of reaching demographic objectives, unlike the one-child policy in China (Greenhalgh 2008) or the "baby bonus" law in Italy, which gave Italian heterosexual parents a monetary bonus if they had a second child (Krause and Marchesi 2007). This emphasis on creating modern citizens who regulate their fertility gives off the illusion that reproduction is just part of a larger development scheme, but in reality, reproduction was framed as one of the major "problems" that needed to be fixed in order for Morocco to move forward and to become a major political and economic player in the global scene. James Ferguson (1990) suggests the key to studying development lies within the relationship between planning and the rationality behind the process by policy makers and officials involved and the actual "intelligibility of outcomes." This relationship is situated within Moroccan women's reproductive bodies. The goal of liberating the body has actually led to increased control over the body as Morocco engages in broader transnational development and political reforms occurring in the MENA.

## DEMOGRAPHIC CONCERNS POST INDEPENDENCE

After independence, the newly minted Moroccan government worked to build a modern nation-state. In 1965, just nine years after independence, the Economic Planning Department published a report that pushed questions of reproduction to the forefront of the government's agenda. Prior to independence, French and Spanish authorities viewed Morocco as underpopulated and allowed thousands of Europeans to settle in the protectorate, particularly under French rule in the 1930s and 1940s (Pennell 2000). In the 1950s, the country started to feel the effects of the foreign settlers. The planning report stated that at the time, population growth was 3.2 percent annually (Brown 1968). In its population projections to 1985, the department argued that Morocco would face numerous economic consequences in the areas of education and employment if the growth rate remained above 3 percent per year. The report suggested that major economic gains could only be made if the rate decreased to 2 percent annually. These projections, coupled with the fact that Morocco's neighbor Tunisia had already implemented a family planning program in 1963, encouraged the government to take action. There is some evidence that representatives from the World Bank encouraged Morocco to adopt the Tunisian model of family planning, and, in 1966, the Moroccan government launched its national family planning program as part of the Ministry of Health, where the program is still housed today.

The family planning program began with the establishment of a national population commission in addition to local commissions; however, the program was not accompanied by policies concerning the legalization of abortion, the accessibility of contraception, or the improvement of women's rights (Maddy-Weitzman 1992). In Morocco, abortion is only permissible when it would save the mother's life or to preserve her physical or mental health, but in all other incidences, such as sexual assault or incest, the procedure is not allowed. Historically Morocco has had one of the highest maternal mortality rates in the MENA even though progress has been made in recent decades. In 1990 the rate was three hundred maternal deaths per one hundred thousand live births, and in 2010 the rate has decreased to an estimated one hundred maternal deaths per one hundred thousand live births (WHO 2012).[3] Even with progress, the concern surrounding unsafe abortions cuts across various sectors of the medical community and government. One of the earliest accomplishments of the family planning program was the abolition in 1967 of a French law that prohibited the advertising and sale of contraception (Ayad and Roudi 2006; see Sargent and Cordell 2003 for more on France's negative attitude towards family planning in its colonies). As part of the program, the government began to open family planning clinics in mainly urban areas. Two "Knowledge, Attitude, and Practice" (KAP) surveys showed that generally men and women in Morocco were in favor of adopting contraceptive methods.

The government started the family planning program with the intention of producing an atmosphere that was conducive to the acceptance of family planning instead of strict physical controls; however, the actual methods by which such an environment was produced included increasing surveillance of women's fertility in the name of building a modern nation. Sociologist and feminist activist Fatima Mernissi (1975) pointed out that Morocco's five-year plan from 1968 to 1972, which aimed to cut the birthrate, was in fact a demographic policy. Although the program was believed to increase people's awareness of family planning and its benefits, thus encouraging them to adopt a method, Mernissi points out that it actually began with the goal of decreasing men and women's fertility. This method was unsuccessful overall. Come 1973, the birthrate was in fact at its highest since independence at 7.4 children per woman (Courbage 1995) and approximately only 3 percent of women in Morocco within childbearing age had adopted contraception.

The spike in fertility after the conclusion of the five-year plan left the Moroccan government unsure how to go about addressing population growth effectively so that it would not equal or exceed the country's economic growth. This was a grave concern raised by development organizations based in the United States and the World Bank. Increasing contraceptive use among women and making reproductive health integral to the public health system were the predominant methods by which the government went about controlling fertility, but medical personnel were not trained properly in family planning or reproductive health (Maddy-Weitzman 1992). At a conference that focused on population in the MENA, scholars and researchers stated that there was no political consensus that supported the institution of "a meaningful population policy" (Calabrese 2001). Right-wing conservatives, Islamic parties, and leftist liberals in Morocco opposed family planning, albeit for different reasons, and therefore the policy "consisted essentially of 'empty political pronouncements and unrealistic targets'" (Calabrese 2001).

Whereas the premise of the family planning program was to foster an environment favorable towards contraceptive use, I make note that demographic targets accompanied such rhetoric. This raises questions as to whether or not allowing women to choose to use contraception was the main objective of the program. This conflation of personal choice and control is a worldwide occurrence. Mary S. Thompson points this out in her study of reproductive politics in Chiapas, Mexico, where "numerical target setting (population control) runs in the face of an informed choice agenda (birth control/reproductive health)" (Russell and Thompson 2000, 12). She "warns about population control masquerading behind an empty rhetoric of 'participation'" (ibid.). In the beginning, the Moroccan program aimed to decrease the crude birthrate from forty-nine to forty-five births per one thousand people, but this goal was not accomplished for numerous, and slightly ambiguous, reasons (Chandrasekaran and Hermalin 1975). In particular, the reigning king, King Hassan II, did not speak about family planning publicly. He even signed the 1966 UN declaration that recognized the severity of unplanned population growth and the importance of family planning to the well-being of parents, children, and the nation as a whole. Although the king supported reproductive health measures in theory, he did not discuss it with the Moroccan public until a speech in 1978 (Grosse 1982).

King Hassan II not addressing reproductive health or family planning publicly for over a decade made garnering and sustaining the attention and support of citizens an extremely challenging task for the Ministry of Health and international development agencies, such as USAID, which worked in Morocco on such matters. Without King Hassan's support early on, the atmosphere that the family planning program intended to create was limited. Therefore, more strain was placed on controlling women's reproduction in order to reach demographic and development objectives. In its infancy, the program actually reproduced the rhetoric of authoritarian control that it attempted to counter, and the rest of this chapter demonstrates that these contradictions and paradoxes continue with more recent neoliberal reforms to development and health policies.

## DEVELOPMENT POLICIES IN MOROCCO

Sketching the transition from economic to social development is crucial for understanding the rise of the family planning program in Morocco and current policies concerning reproductive healthcare. Women's reproductive bodies are at the center of this transition in the development agenda as Morocco tries to create an international image for itself based on the modernization process and improvements in women's rights. However, the coming of an agenda based on social rather than economic development also brought greater control, albeit indirect control, over women's bodies as they need to adhere to certain childbearing and childrearing practices in order to be considered modernized Moroccan citizens. In the years directly following independence from France, the Moroccan government focused on domestic, economic, and social policy under the reign of King Mohammed V, but upon his passing in 1961, his son, King Hassan II, took over the process of building the independent nation-state. The government followed the dominant development agenda at the time, "believing only economic growth would bring about improvement in social indicators. Yet, simply following the basic rules of development did not lead to sustained economic growth or sufficient human capital and industrialization to become competitive in the world economy" (Cohen and Jaidi 2006, 35). These challenges to development became hotly debated topics between state officials and international development agencies.

The postindependence years in Morocco were in reality anything but hopeful for many. Termed *al-sanawat al-sawda* in Arabic and *les années de plomb* in French (translated as "the black years" or "the years of lead"), nation building postindependence is described as a somber and fearful time. Hundreds of people seen in opposition to King Hassan's regime were taken as political prisoners, and many people who spoke out against the corruptness of the government disappeared (Slyomovics 2001). After a failed coup attempt in the 1970s, anyone opposed to the regime was viewed as a threat to the throne. However, in the early 1990s, massive shifts began to occur in the country's policies. King Hassan II stated that he would "turn the page indefinitively" (quoted in Slyomovics 2001) in order to address the political prisoner situation. Just a few years earlier, he created an advisory council on human rights with various subgroups organized to investigate crimes against humanity, and in 1993 the Ministry of Human Rights was formed.

In the midst of turning its attention to human rights and focusing on protecting and preserving citizens' lives, the Moroccan government realized that economic development ultimately failed in the country because social indicators (healthcare, illiteracy, poverty, and education, for instance) were still not at the levels the government intended. Social development, particularly in the late 1990s after international conferences on the relationship between women's rights and development, became a more pressing issue.

From the mid-1990s onward, social development, policy making, and institutional reform became major topics in government and civic debates. Most notably, the International Conference on Population and Development (ICPD) that took place in 1994 in Cairo, Egypt, had a tremendous impact on development policies, women's rights, and reproductive health programs in Morocco given that it participated in the conference and the development of its Plan of Action. Mrs. Abdellah, a feminist activist and longtime staff member at the UNFPA office in Rabat, explained to me, "The ICPD in 1994 was very important for reproductive health in Morocco; 1994 was a year of change here." The report for the ICPD begins with:

> The 1994 International Conference on Population and Development occurs at a defining moment in the history of international cooperation. With the growing recognition of global population, development and environmental interdependence, the opportunity to adopt suitable macro- and socio-economic policies to promote sustained economic growth in the context of sustainable development in all countries and to mobilize human and financial resources for global problem- solving has never been greater. (UN 1994)

The ICPD report goes on to state:

> Over the past 20 years, many parts of the world have undergone remarkable demographic, social, economic, environmental and political change. Many countries have made substantial progress in expanding access to reproductive health care and lowering birth rates, as well as in lowering death rates and raising education and income levels, including the educational and economic status of women. While the advances of the past two decades in areas such as increased use of contraception, decreased maternal mortality, implemented sustainable development plans and projects and enhanced educational programmes provide a basis for optimism about successful implementation of the present Programme of Action, much remains to be accomplished. (Ibid.)

The International Monetary Fund (IMF) views Morocco as a success story because of structural adjustment programs that took place in the 1980s; however, at the same time, the World Bank has criticized the country for not being more proactive in terms of social development (Cohen and Jaidi 2006). These international criticisms prompted the country's participation in the ICPD and its subsequent Plan of Action, which goals included implementing programs that focus on both social issues and development simultaneously as they cannot be considered separate from one another. They also encouraged the Moroccan government to make improving citizens' lives—in particular women—a top political priority. In 1999, with the death of King Hassan II, his son, King Mohammed VI, took the throne. With King Mohammed VI came a new regime of government that focuses on creating democracy within the country.[4] He has been called many names, such as "Morocco's first feminist king" and the "king of the poor." In a television address right after taking the throne, he promised to tackle issues of corruption in the government, to alleviate poverty in Morocco, and to further investigate human rights abuses. In his early years of ruling, he said, "Moroccans want a strong monarchy, one that is democratic and executive" (quoted in Cohen and Jaidi 2006, 1). King Mohammed VI continued in his speech, "In Morocco, the King is not content to reign. I reign and I work with my government in a clear constitutional framework that defines the responsibility of each."[5] In a royal speech in 2005, the king emphasized the country's movement towards modernity in order to promote democratic values: "We have worked without relent on reaffirming a state of law and institutions, promoting *the values of responsible citizenship*, the modernization of the economy, and the concretization of the spirit of solidarity, all for assuring the practice of a democracy with all of *its social and human benefit*" (italics added).[6]

Within a relatively short period of time, from 1956 to the late 1990s, there was a massive regime shift in Morocco from a strong and central monarchy to a discourse of democracy, privatization, and responsible citizenship that would come to penetrate nearly every domain of life, including reproduction. Nikolas Rose and Peter Miller have noted, "Within this new regime of the actively responsible self, individuals are to fulfill their national obligations not through their relations of dependency and obligation to one another, but through seeking to fulfill themselves within a variety of micro-moral domains or 'communities'—families, workplaces, schools, leisure associations, neighbourhoods" (2008, 214). The transition from a welfare state to individual responsibility that Rose and Miller point out is a hallmark in transnational development trends, with which Morocco is intimately engaged. Cameron Khosrowshahi writes, "A successful privatization effort has heralded Morocco's formal break with the *dirigiste* economic policies of the past in favor of the disengagement of the state from certain social and economic obligations" (1997, 242). Khosrowshahi goes on to suggest that privatization actually has done very little to "empower new groups" in Morocco or to reduce the wealth disparities between classes. Whereas he is directly addressing economic policies, I argue that rhetoric of privatization has been expanded to reproduction in part because the state recognized that it was not able to decrease the TFR or to expand reproductive health services alone. Partnerships with private organizations and the promotion of responsible citizenship rhetoric (although done under the pretense of improving the health system and creating an environment that is conducive to the acceptance of family planning) were necessary to incorporating women's reproductive bodies into the state's agenda for modernization.

## THE RELATIONSHIP BETWEEN PRIVATE ORGANIZATIONS AND THE STATE

The RHO in Morocco has a long history with the state, furthering the argument in the social sciences that the practices, policies, and objectives of NGOs and IOs must be analyzed within the same frame as the state (Elyachar 2005). In the 1970s and the 1980s, Morocco experienced economic hardship due to the decline of the price in its exports. Morocco monopolizes the phosphate industry.[7] The price of phosphates declined dramatically, which meant that the Moroccan government could not subsidize as many amenities for citizens as it had in the past. In response to these economic tough times, the government improved its family planning program so that the population could be more manageable given the country's financial resources. International agencies including USAID and the International Planned Parenthood Federation (IPPF) began investing large sums of money into reproductive health programs in the country, although by the 1980s, USAID had pulled out of healthcare in Morocco and invested its funds into governance and education projects, most notably women's literacy and girls' education programs.[8] Before funding was reorganized, USAID money was given to help Morocco set up programs in order to expand the voluntary use of contraception and to enhance "population and demographic planning" (Maddy-Weitzman 1992, 74). Instead of a holistic approach to reproductive health that integrates such services into the public health system, USAID influenced the Moroccan government to focus on decreasing the TFR to create a more manageable population.[9]

The RHO was established with the intent of providing sexual and reproductive health services to men and women despite their age, marital status, ethnicity, or residence. Mernissi (1975) suggests that the key to a successful family planning program in Morocco is to make medical services attractive to citizens, much more so than they had been previously. The family planning program and the RHO tried to do just that. Dr. Binjal explained that he and the board faced a conundrum while establishing the organization. A few years after its formation, Dr. Binjal left the organization to pursue a career in various international health organizations, including the IPPF, which describes itself as a "a global provider and a leading advocate of sexual and reproductive health and rights for all,"[10] and he is now a well-respected academic and activist in Morocco. Whereas the organization aims to improve access to sexual and reproductive health services and education for all citizens, the public health system has been known to make it difficult for adolescents and unmarried men and women to receive services and information given that sexual relations outside of marriage (in addition to adultery) are prohibited by Islam.[11]

At the time of its establishment, there was a political backlash against the left in Morocco, with events like the disappearance of Mehdi Ben Barka, the former leader of the leftist party *L'Union Nationale des Forces Populaires.*[12] The *Istiqlāl* party, a more conservative political party in Morocco that held the majority of Parliament seats until 2011, led the struggle for independence from France, but it was in opposition to practices such as family planning because it could disrupt the structure of the familial unit and of society.[13] The *Istiqlāl* party opposed family planning on both religious and nationalist grounds. The party founder, Allal al-Fassi, could not comprehend why Muslims would want to limit the size of their communities by having fewer children. According to him, decreasing population growth would only weaken Morocco, a newly independent nation-state that was carving out a niche for itself in the Arab world. The party claimed that contraception was merely a "Western" tactic to impede the development of emerging "Third-World" nations and that citizens should not adopt family planning no matter what the costs may be (Maddy-Weitzman 1992).

The RHO was established in an attempt to counter the notion that reproductive healthcare was a Western strategy to influence the development of the non-West. The RHO has adapted strategies, objectives, and international standards concerning sexual and reproductive healthcare in order to fit the particular conditions and circumstances under which it works. There are five domains the RHO targets within its specific social context: access, abortion, advocacy, adolescents, and AIDS (HIV). Some liberal political activists in Morocco have criticized the organization for not being progressive enough and, therefore, have actually reinscribed notions that women are to be thought of as citizens and as humans through their biology. In other words, the RHO has not focused on women's empowerment or gender equality enough through their campaigns and programs, but rather their bodies. The organization works with private and public sectors to increase knowledge about and use of contraceptives and to provide information to communities about sexual and reproductive health. It aims to consistently offer high-quality medical care to its patients.[14] The RHO health clinics around Morocco are in large cities and smaller towns. There are mobile units that travel to rural areas to distribute birth control (the pill and condoms) and information; a few health centers that provide services to adolescents;[15] and nearly eight hundred community volunteers that provide training to citizens about personal hygiene, reproductive and sexual health, and healthcare in general. All services in the clinics and the outreach supplies cost a small fee, which is used to sustain the organization and its staff. These prices, however, are much less than what men and women would pay at a private doctor or hospital for services or at a pharmacy for contraception.

In our interview, Dr. Binjal said, "The [RHO] has missed two major opportunities to make a difference in my opinion: HIV/AIDS and poverty. The [international] goals are very progressive, but in Morocco, the [organization] has not implemented them as quickly as they could have." The RHO was in part created because of the failure of the five-year plan (1968–1972) to decrease the TFR and because of the pressure from outside Morocco to address reproductive health issues. But Dr. Binjal's quote indicates that the goals of the organization have expanded far beyond just family planning and controlling the TFR and population growth rate. This can only be accomplished through addressing social matters, such as poverty and STDs. Hajjer, an executive staff member at the RHO who has worked there since the early 1990s in finance, stated that even in the time that she has been there, "the goals of the [organization] have changed. We focus on sexual and reproductive health but it is not just about women and their bodies anymore. It is about society. The goals have expanded and become much broader." When I asked why the organization has expanded the scope of its work beyond just providing contraception, Hajjer responded that it is due to the demands of Moroccan society and the healthcare system. Through disseminating information to the public and offering medical services to everyone, despite their age, marital status, or ability to pay, the RHO has always intended to open up a nationwide dialogue about sexuality, fertility, pregnancy, and abortion in addition to a conversation about their relevance to other social issues, including illiteracy, education, and poverty.

However, I question whether or not the RHO prioritizes the needs of Moroccans or improvements in social services and infrastructure over the government's need to survey and control women's reproductive bodies. I play the devil's advocate here for a moment because the institutionalization of an NGO is "a double-edged sword" in Morocco, as it is elsewhere in the world. In Morocco, the NGO must work within state power and be recognized by the government, which is a long and tedious process.[16] The NGO must adhere to the state's overarching policies, but, at the same time, it must be independent enough to tackle issues that the state might not otherwise. It needs to have enough leeway to fill in gaps. For the RHO, this includes addressing the sexual and reproductive health needs of individuals in rural areas and of those who are not married. But Dr. Binjal reminded me that this can become extremely dangerous because if the government relies too much on the institution to accomplish these particular tasks, then it will not be held accountable by national and international entities if certain health goals are not met. The RHO, like other NGOs, straddles a very fine line so that it can deliver services adequately but yet not take on complete responsibility for them. He explained to me in our interview, "An NGO is a double-edged sword. The government cannot give complete control to the NGO because then it will not take any responsibility when something goes wrong, but the government needs the organization to address health needs. If the government is not involved at all, then there will be a disaster."

Development reports from a five-year period (2005 to 2010) demonstrate that controlling women's reproduction is the stepping-stone for development because in theory a lower birthrate will allow for financial and material resources to be better distributed. Dr. Binjal's comments in regards to the RHO's missed chances to address poverty and HIV/AIDS points to its continued work in this type of framework—it prioritized providing contraception and other services to women over addressing social and public health concerns. Julia Elyachar has masterfully demonstrated that in many cases, "the state is not an adequate unit of analysis . . . instead practices carried out by diverse institutional forms, such as the state, IOs, and NGOs, need to be studied together in one field of power" (2005, 29). What is of interest for me is Elyachar's theorization of the state and civil society as entangled modes of governance. I am not discounting the RHO's goals of empowering women or improving reproductive health services, but rather I am pointing out alternative modes for being for women that are created in a society that focuses on their reproductive labor as a primary way for them to be incorporated into the development scheme.

## HEALTH POLICIES AND WOMEN'S BODIES POST–CAIRO CONFERENCE

In the five target domains of the RHO, bodily practices, especially those of women, are at each of their centers despite the fact that the organization works in a much wider framework for development. There is a slippage back into the language of biological reproduction, which has caused me to question the organization's main premises. I am not attempting to create a binary of good policies and programs versus bad policies and programs; instead, I offer an alternative view that highlights the unintended consequences of the adoption of such an agenda. Before the ICPD in 1994, as Hajjer mentioned, the RHO worked specifically on family planning and reproductive health issues. After, its goals were expanded to meet the changing needs of Moroccans and newer global health standards that focused on incorporating reproduction into social development. Susan Cohen and Cory Richards emphasize the worldwide shift in development that took place after the ICPD:

> The 1994 International Conference on Population and Development (ICPD), the United Nation's third decennial conference on population issues, marked a milestone in population policy and politics. It achieved worldwide consensus that population is a top-ranking issue worthy of consideration at the highest level of all governments; it placed the discussion of population firmly in a development context; and it identified women and their status as central to sustaining global development efforts. (1994, 272)

Population has long been a concern for Morocco, even before the ICPD. The ICPD action plan urged the government, along with other governments from around the world, to integrate population into development agendas. This actually makes the paradox even stronger given that the reproductive body was just supposed to be one part of the development plan, with other important social issues such as women's empowerment being addressed. But the reproductive body actually remained firmly at the center despite the broader social development agenda and the targeted domains of the RHO.[17]

## Adolescents

Young male and female reproductive bodies are key to the broader discussion that the RHO is trying to open up in Morocco. The RHO incorporates individuals into its agenda who tend to be marginalized in reproductive healthcare, including youth and poorer men and women. There are active youth groups run through the RHO comprised of young men and women between fourteen and twenty-four years old. Every summer the organization sponsors a youth festival that uses creativity to promote positive messages about sexual and reproductive health. For instance, in 2008 the festival took place in a seaside town about an hour south of Rabat. Nearly three hundred young men and women gathered for three days. The festival centered on a music competition where each youth group was required to sing a song of any genre they like about an aspect of HIV/AIDS (transmission, prevention, stigmatization) in Arabic, French, or an Amazigh dialect.[18] The leader of the festival is a young man named Ali, who is in his midtwenties and also worked with the Ministry of Youth. Ali had been a longtime member of the council before he took the position as leader. He spoke harshly of the government at the festival, charging that it did not provide young people with adequate education about sexual and reproductive health, disease, or medical services that are available. Ali made the body central to his criticisms because he claimed that youth do not know as much about their bodies as they should. He highlighted that the central nature of the reproductive body to modernization is created through interactions between policies, medical practices, and individual beliefs. In addition, every summer the RHO's youth groups in Rabat and in the southern coastal town of Agadir put on a Caravan in August. Over the course of a few weeks, the youth periodically go to the beach to talk with children, other youth, and adults about health concerns. They discuss sexual and reproductive health, such as where is the organization's closest clinic and ways to prevent unwanted pregnancies, as well as more common health concerns like personal hygiene, smoking, and the need for physical exercise. Prior to the Caravan, the youth participate in extensive training sessions so that they are up-to-date on the latest health information. I attended one session in Rabat where a doctor, staff from the Ministry of Health, and Ali led a two-day workshop to discuss the proper ways to approach people on the beach, the types of vocabulary they should use so that they could be understood by everyone in the public, and how to encourage parents to talk to their children about pressing health issues. The main theme of this workshop was that the youth must provide accurate information to individuals of all ages about the issues that affect their bodies, meaning they were not supposed to speak to a very young girl about preventing pregnancy; rather they should talk to her about common hygiene issues. The types of information they needed to discuss would be different because they are at different life stages. The leaders stressed that speaking to an older adult male is vastly different than speaking to a teenage girl. The types of health information to be disseminated are to be gauged by the recipient's current bodily practices.

Young men and women in Agadir received similar training in the summer of 2008. At this workshop, the leaders emphasized youth today do not understand their bodies in part because of differing vocabularies. Mara, a woman in her thirties who oversaw the youth group in this region, led many of the sessions. She explained to me that these young men and women do not often receive this information in Moroccan Arabic. She stated, "This is not common. This session does not always happen. They may receive this information in school, but it is in French. Do they speak to each other in French? No, they talk in Arabic or *Tamazight* every day. If they cannot speak about their health or their bodies or the clinics in general because they do not have the words, then nothing will change." At this particular training event, eighteen youth gathered at the RHO clinic in Agadir to talk about the best ways to change people's attitudes towards sexual and reproductive health and to lift societal taboos that exist around the subject. The last day even included goal setting for 2008 and 2009 with Mr. Masjeel, the executive director of the RHO, and Mr. Benbellah, the finance director. What is striking is that Mara's statement about language and the body makes sessions like these even more crucial for youth and modernization efforts in the country because this type of training is able to equip young men and women—the future generations—with the vocabularies to discuss bodily practices and other issues surrounding the body with their peers and to make better decisions about their reproductive bodies.[19]

## Access

Access to quality reproductive health services for everyone is one of the main focuses for the RHO. The organization's strategic plan states that poorer men and women are marginalized and face discrimination in terms of access to family planning and reproductive healthcare, but underneath this statement is the assumption that if working-class men and women do not have access to such services, then being able to regulate their fertility and to have healthy pregnancies would be extremely difficult. Therefore, they could not control their fertility and make informed choices about their reproductive practices and thus could not become the modern accountable citizens that the Moroccan government intends to create. Socioeconomic obstacles in combination with limited access leave such individuals with fewer choices when it comes to finding reproductive health services. The

RHO intends to improve its ability to provide contraception and education through its numerous clinics around Morocco and community-based programs in poorer quarters of cities, smaller towns, and rural regions. The main objective of these programs, according to the strategic plan, is to provide individuals and communities a sense of responsibility, especially the poor, marginalized, and underserved, so they are able to make informed decisions about their bodies and their sexual and reproductive health.

These community-based efforts rely upon volunteers. The volunteers are male and female shopkeepers, merchants, housewives, and mothers who receive training from the RHO. They are then put in charge of taking orders for and distributing contraception to local individuals. A number of volunteers work for smaller private community health clinics throughout the country. The volunteers visit homes of community members or hold focus groups in order to discuss reproductive health as well as general health concerns, including what to do if complications arise during pregnancy or childbirth and proper ways to use various contraceptive methods. They also make individuals aware of the RHO and its clinics, which serve anyone despite age, ethnicity, class, or marital status. (The RHO has a few clinics dedicated to just healthcare for adolescents.) A twenty-six-year-old volunteer named Badrdine owns a clothing store in a small town outside of Rabat and has worked for the RHO for three years. When I asked about who he sells supplies to, he responded, "I sell the condoms to teenage boys who live in towns close to here. I sell a lot of them. I keep one dirham from every sale." A second female volunteer who works at a small clinic in the same town as where Badrdine lives stated that young boys do purchase condoms from her, but, most often, they are not from the local area. They are frightened by the possibility that someone may see them doing so. Although strides are being made in Morocco by organizations like the RHO, negative social connotations surrounding sexual relations outside of marriage create disparities in access to health services. This exemplifies the argument put forth by Nguyen and Peschard (2003) that much of the work in public health discounts factors other than poverty that create disparities in health services. This poses challenges to the organization in its attempts to reach poorer unmarried men and women (i.e., adolescents) in particular, whose bodies have been framed as the very ones needing to be controlled and conditioned by the state so that there is not a "population bomb" (Ehrlich 1968) in the future.

## Advocacy

In order to successfully carry out programs, the RHO has worked through the method of Information, Education, and Communication (IEC) since its establishment. In the strategic plan and other planning documents of the organization, the French verbs *améliorer* (improve), *renforcer* (reinforce), *sensibiliser* (to increase public awareness), and *responsabiliser* (to make responsible, to promote) appear quite frequently. These verbs lend themselves to the creation of an environment where reproductive health services are widely available, accepted by the overall public, and framed as a way to achieve improved personal well-being. In short, this is an environment where citizens self-govern themselves. According to these documents, the organization does not work through direct bodily intervention or strict policies, but instead offers men and women the tools they need to make the best decisions about fertility, their bodies, and their overall health. Whereas administration, volunteers, and staff in its clinics provide the information to beneficiaries, it is up to individuals to make the "right" choices, which are defined primarily by social development discourses and ideologies. IEC actually problematizes the role of intervention in family planning because it creates a contradiction for many women. Conflicts between cultural values in Morocco that make family and childbearing a critical part of a woman's life and neoliberal logic that reshape their sense of self may actually complicate their choices about their bodies. In this framework, choosing not to use contraception or not to use the available reproductive health services is erased from the options in which they are to choose from.

Hajjer, the executive staff member at the RHO who I discussed previously in this chapter, believes that the organization continues to try to improve sexual and reproductive healthcare for all citizens, but the methods by which the organization goes about doing this in the time in which she has been there have changed dramatically. IEC has been broadened in order to address various domains other than family planning: maternal healthcare, pregnancy, childbirth, and infant health, just to name a few. In the 1970s and 1980s, the government was mainly concerned about a possible population explosion due to the high fertility rate, the elevated population growth rate, and the low rate of contraceptive use. It was within this climate that the RHO was formed. However, now that other reproductive health issues have been identified as possibly hindering Morocco's development—maternal mortality and poor maternal healthcare, for example—the RHO has adapted to these changes and taken on such concerns through advocating for policy changes within the government itself. Keeping this in mind, the next section of this chapter analyzes the changes in development policies that have sparked adjustments in the organization's programs and gives a better sense of the political and cultural milieu that the organization operates within today given that it was key to my ethnographic fieldwork.

## CHANGING REGIMES, CHANGING POLICY: RETRACING THE BODY IN DEVELOPMENT IN MOROCCO

In the years immediately following Morocco's independence from France in 1956, King Mohammed V, the father of King Hassan II, implemented a modernizing monarchy. Whereas the language is the same as is being used today, *modernité*, the meaning was much different. King Mohammed V, who was the Sultan of Morocco from 1927 to 1953 and then took the title of king from 1957 to 1961 after being exiled to Corsica and Madagascar by the French prior to independence, exercised a very active political role. Modernizing in this sense was dictated by not allowing radical groups to overthrow the order of the new nation-state through implementing laws like the Personal Status Code (*Moudawana*) that brought everyone's bodies under one regime. King Hassan II, upon taking the throne after his death, established an authoritative regime in the country. Although he drafted a constitution with the intention of moving towards more global definitions of modernity, the document in reality gave him sole authority in the government.[20] Modernization has shifted in its goals from building a unified nation-state to equal political representation to, finally, democracy and individual participation today. At each of these stages, however, bodily practices have been a key concern for the government. In Morocco, there has always been a fear within the government of upheaval and rebellion from various ethnic and religious groups as well as social classes (Cohen 2004). In order to quell this, the human body, and particularly women's bodies, has been kept at the center of development policies and politics.

Even with privatization in the realm of health in the 1980s and 1990s, and partnerships with organizations like the RHO and international development agencies, government officials in Morocco debated as to why economic reforms did not particularly lead to increased economic growth or, more importantly, to improved social indicators. Modernization, in these terms, focused on economics with the belief that they would lead to improvements within society. Subsequently, the Moroccan state shifted its main focus from economic development to social development come the mid-1990s, shortly after the ICPD and the Fourth World Conference on Women held in Beijing in 1995: "the ICPD Programme of Action consolidated the shift in population policies and programmes from reliance on demographic targets and compulsory family planning services to a rights-based approach, based on reproductive health choices" (Sinding and Bouzidi 2002, 323). Women became central to discourses of development not just in Morocco but worldwide as money was funneled into projects dealing with issues pertinent to women's lives, such as reproductive and maternal health. The Moroccan government turned its attention to bringing together strategies for economic growth and for enhancing the lives of citizens at the same time. One of the main objectives became the creation of "modern" and responsible citizens. King Mohammed VI is quoted as stating in a speech in 2005 that Moroccans themselves must be willing to make "responsible choices" as to their everyday lives and must be prepared to become "modernized" citizens.[21] The government argued that men and women need to make conscious decisions that will not only improve their well-being, but will enhance the nation's progress and help the country become a major player in the world economy (Zemni and Bogaert 2009).

Whereas it can be argued that this shift in development was a political move, it coincided with a change of the country's ruling powers. Since ascending to power, King Mohammed VI has been applauded for his attention to and advocating for the poor and women; a 2007 article in *Forbes* estimated his worth at $2 billion due to phosphates but hailed him for choosing to discuss more pressing social issues in public rather than exports.[22] His wedding to Lalla Salma Bennani, a former engineer at the industrial firm Omnium Nord Africain (ONA), was the first royal wedding to a nonroyal in the country's history and was widely photographed. (No one saw photos or portraits of the king's mother until after the passing of King Hassan II.) He even granted her a royal title. To me, this is a crucial piece of the puzzle because the rapid change in Morocco in the realm of women's rights is intimately connected with the king's break away from marriage customs of past royals. Many in Morocco assumed that this was a sign of public commitment he made upon taking the throne to work on women's issues and poverty. What is interesting here, however, is that Princess Lalla Salma's body—photographs of her wedding day, pictures of what she is wearing, and the king's control (or lack thereof) over her actions—is at the center of people's curiosity and the debate about the royal family.[23]

King Mohammed VI is viewed as being much more open to reform than his late father. In 2002, he made the voting age eighteen instead of twenty to allow "the Moroccan youth to overwhelmingly join our project of a modern, democratic society."[24] In addition, women have been guaranteed to hold at least thirty seats in the Parliament, roughly 10 percent of the total number of seats.[25] And most importantly, the king has tried to make development a participatory process. This is in theory rather than practice as problems still remain concerning what participation really means; although he has publicly stated that he has taken the advice of feminist groups and human rights activists under serious consideration, which has produced projects such as changes to religious education to remove photos and discussion of the veil from school textbooks and the prosecution of human rights abuses.

Civil society has become crucial to the government's endeavors of creating "modernized" citizens who lead a modern nation-state. Modernity under King Mohammed VI means democracy as well as participation at the national and individual levels. In 2005, in a speech to the United Nations General Assembly, the king stated that the goal of the government is to "free large segments of the population . . . from the yoke of poverty, illiteracy and unemployment, thus enabling them to lead the decent life we wish to offer all our citizens."[26] The objective for the current regime is not only to create a democratic Morocco where Islamic extremism is barred and women's rights are paramount, but to produce citizens' minds and bodies that will be able to handle the responsibilities that accompany democracy and will be able to recognize and take advantage of the resources provided to them by the private and public sectors. Rose (2000) critiques policy makers who claim that this type of politics is new. He argues that whereas this shift to "moral subjects" and "responsible citizens" has taken place for years, lawmakers in the United States and Europe in recent decades have called it a "novel form of politics." In reference to the nineteenth century, he writes, "Like that earlier project, the current Third Way claims to be more than merely a middle road defined by what it avoids. It aspires to be nothing less than a founding set of moral beliefs for a new politics" (2000, 1396). The fact that Morocco has engaged with such a logic in the last two decades destabilizes Rose's assumption that these are "Western" subjects (see Greenhalgh 2009 for another example), and it makes Islam, along with the politics surrounding the religion, a key driver in the production of these citizens.

## THE LAUNCH OF THE NATIONAL INITIATIVE FOR HUMAN DEVELOPMENT IN 2005

Women's reproductive bodies are the foundation of the current development initiative in Morocco, the INDH. Their productive and economic labors are given less importance than their abilities to control the fertility rate and raise the future generations of citizens. This frames women as citizens through their bodies and their bodily practices, particularly those related to childbearing and childrearing. I stress that I am not attempting to make this a binary of positive and negative change. Instead, I delineate the unintended consequences and side effects of the current development policy, which are neither "good nor bad" but are creating new ways for Moroccan women to think of themselves as women, mothers, and citizens, as well as new gendered meanings of development. Norma Alarcón, Caren Kaplan, and Minoo Moallem argue that nation-states often participate in the "institutionalization of women's subordination by means of regulatory processes, the discursive formations that construct and discipline citizen-subjects" (1999, 12). Through current discourses of human development and responsible citizenship and through the reliance on civil society in the domains of health and women's rights, including the RHO, the Moroccan government is actively disciplining women to be a particular type of "modern" citizen who is largely connected with her reproductive body, even though the rhetoric behind this is focused on holistic well-being (i.e. financially, family, and the nation).

The INDH is an important initiative that puts Morocco's "social issues at the forefront of the country's political priorities" (Martín 2006, 1). Whereas the initiative has targeted specific geographic areas and groups—most notably women and the poor—I focus here on the ways that the message of responsibility and self-governance that is being conveyed impacts daily life in the realms of reproduction, gender, health, and motherhood. The government has publicly recognized social problems are the primary challenge to development, not economic growth. In another speech to the

Parliament, King Mohammed VI stated that the government will undertake "'social modernization' through integrated public policies," and at the same time it will acknowledge the "importance of public participation" (Martín 2006, 2). The king emphasized the need to build a network of associations, international and local development agencies, and government offices for his vision of development to succeed.

The INDH mobilizes the country's institutional and financial resources, both domestic and international, to improve the population's living conditions and the social indicators. The three main objectives of the initiative are: to increase income-generating activities, to improve infrastructure and social services (healthcare, education, literacy, poverty), and to provide assistance to the most vulnerable groups in Morocco identified by the government (women, the poor, and adolescents). It is imperative to understand the genealogy of human development, a concept that has come to dominate development today around the globe. Human development was commissioned by the UNDP, which developed the Human Development Index (HDI) in 1990. Human development encompasses much more than just the growth or decline of people's incomes; it is concerned with creating

*Table 1.1* Select 2011 Inequality-Adjusted HDI Rankings

| Country | Rank | HDI Value |
|---|---|---|
| | *Very High Human Development* | |
| Norway | 1 | 0.943 |
| United States | 4 | 0.910 |
| Qatar | 37 | 0.831 |
| | *High Human Development* | |
| Uruguay | 48 | 0.783 |
| Saudi Arabia | 56 | 0.770 |
| Lebanon | 71 | 0.739 |
| | *Medium Human Development* | |
| Egypt | 113 | 0.644 |
| **Morocco** | **130** | **0.582** |
| Ghana | 135 | 0.541 |
| | *Low Human Development* | |
| Pakistan | 145 | 0.504 |
| Yemen | 154 | 0.462 |
| Democratic Republic of the Congo | 187 | 0.286 |

*Source:* Adapted from UNDP (2011).

an environment in which people can easily "develop their full potential and lead productive, creative lives in accord with their needs and interests."[27] In this sense, economic growth is only a means of expanding the range of people's choices and freedoms.

Central to human development is the enhancement of human capabilities. According to the UNDP, the most basic capacities by which the HDI is measured are: living a long and healthy life, being educated and knowledgeable, and having a decent standard of living. This framing of development and individuals' lives is certainly not novel to political theory (Arendt 1958; Nussbaum 2001), but, rather, it is often forgotten in the immediate concern of wealth and resource accumulation.[28] What is striking is that the main objective of the HDI places people back at the center of development by assessing their long-term well-being, in part through mathematical equations and statistical formulas that comprise the index, but they are not the primary concern. In 2004, Morocco ranked 125th out of 177 countries on the HDI; in 2009, it ranked 130th out of 182 countries. In 2011, it ranked 130th out of 187 countries. On all occasions, it was categorized as having "medium human development."

HDI is an alternative to assessing development using gross national product (GNP) or household income, and Morocco has basically taken this quantitative measure and turned it into a qualitative policy that impacts social domains and, most importantly, people's lives and bodies. Mahbub ul Haq, a Pakistani economist and former finance minister who helped develop the HDI, stated, "People often value achievements that do not show up at all, or not immediately, in income or growth figures . . . The objective of development is to create an enabling environment for people to enjoy long, healthy, and creative lives."[29] Amartya Sen, the codeveloper of the index, writes in his book *Development as Freedom*, "Freedoms are not only the primary ends of development, they are also among its principle means . . . Freedoms of different kinds can strengthen one another" (1999, 10–11). Development happens when "unfreedoms" are removed, and, in the case of Morocco, these include poverty, lack of infrastructure, gender inequality, and disparities in education and health services. The notion of "freedom" put forth by Sen and the Moroccan government reaches far beyond increasing technology transfer and expanding economic growth. Rather, such enhancements serve as instruments to facilitate successful development projects, where the end product is the improvement of people's lives and their conditions of existence.

I question whether or not "freedom" in the sense of autonomy and individual choice is even possible for the Moroccan women with whom I worked and whether or not the promotion of "freedom" is masking another predetermined goal set by the government. Given Sen's articulation and the logic of the UNDP about the HDI, human development shares a common vision with human rights (Engle-Merry 2006; Schaft 2010). According to King Mohammed VI in his speech to the UN in 2005, people must be free to exercise their right to choose to actively participate in the decision making that affects their daily lives and well-being. Sen writes, "In general, the consequences of having and exercising a right must ultimately have some bearing on the overall acceptability of that right" (1999, 213). It might be implausible to discuss development without assessing the fulfillment and violation of human liberties as human development requires that individual freedom become a social commitment. However, full control over the body and the ability to exercise one's choices over reproductive decisions and practices are very difficult for many Moroccan women given the complex social and familial networks in which they live. Within the context of patrilocal households, this notion of "freedom" needs to be reconfigured in order to make sense in women's daily lives.

## WOMEN'S INVOLVEMENT IN DEVELOPMENT: CENTERING THE REPRODUCTIVE BODY

Scholarship demonstrates that everyone does not experience development in the same way (Bernal 1997; Ferguson 1990; Unnithan and Srivastava 1997). Dorothy Hodgson asks, "These ambiguities of meaning enable related mystification over the purpose objectives and effects of development. Development for whom? By whom? Toward what goals?" (2001, 8). Historically in Morocco, women have been excluded from "the human" in human development. To emphasize this point, I repeat a quote (first discussed in the introduction) from the report *50 Ans de Développement Humain et Perspectives 2025*, "Thanks to the changes in matrimonial and procreative behaviors of Moroccan women . . . and family planning programs in which a large portion of the female population participated, the country was able to manage the development of its population" (Royaume du Maroc 2006, 8). There is no denying that this quote locates women's roles in development within their abilities to control population growth by regulating their fertility. Their participation and their citizenship are hinged upon this biological fact, even though not all women are even able to have children. Moroccan women are being incorporated into development mainly through their reproductive bodies, but they continuously readapt and reinterpret this logic. This in turn encourages the government, medical community, and development agencies to question their own agendas and tactics. Whereas the development report circumscribes women to their bodies, women are actually active agents in this process rather than passive objects whose bodies just lie in waiting for the development policy and rhetoric to be etched.

*50 Ans de Développement Humain* acknowledges that women have been a "forgotten element" in development in Morocco, particularly since the country achieved independence in 1956. But, the report goes on to say that today women are recognized as key actors in the modernization process. The report states, "Women have played an important role in the evolution of the human potential of independent Morocco. After a period of being the most forgotten element in the human development process, women struggled and have achieved advancements which are now universally recognized" (2006, 11). Moroccan women have been on the periphery of development, even though they have always played key roles in the process. It was not until the publication of this report, and with the recent turn to social development after the ICPD, that women have been recognized as central to the concept of human development in the country and to the production of "modern" Moroccan citizens. In recent decades, there has been a massive global shift of resources into women's organizations and into projects concerning women. Women have become the main targets of many human development initiatives, especially in the Middle East, where humanitarian efforts have remained high in particular in war-torn areas (Abu-Lughod 2002; Jabbra and Jabbra 1992; Mohanty 2003).

Even though the government has realized that women in Morocco play critical and legitimate roles in development, their participation is regulated primarily to the realm of bodily practice. The development report demonstrates that women are considered essential to development through their reproductive bodies more so than their productive labor. The Moroccan population can progress and be better managed only by controlling women's reproductive behaviors through medical practices, such as family planning and maternal healthcare. Historically, the Moroccan government has set up a reciprocal link between women's reproduction and development; development can only occur once population growth and fertility are regulated and once maternal and infant mortality rates have decreased. However, in recent years, since the shift to social development, the rhetoric of development has served as the primary means through which these health concerns will be addressed (and resolved). Through the promotion of responsible citizenship (including having smaller families, seeking prenatal care, and ensuring infant health) the government attempts to improve such social indicators.

Development has brought about great uncertainty among working-class women in Morocco. Rahma Bourqia conducted a study among rural women and discovered that "the most important investment and capital for women is to have children" (1995, 14). This means that accepting family planning can be extremely disruptive to some women's lives in Morocco. Decision making about fertility and childrearing is not purely driven by economic considerations, but it is informed by social and cultural meanings of motherhood, the family, and femininity. Bourqia suggests women are not apt to adopt contraception because having children gives them a role within the family and because their reproductive functions generally strengthen their status in the community. In addition, she argues that giving birth actually defines their existence as women and wives both socially and psychologically. Adopting contraception comes with "social costs," some of which are too great for women to bear.

In a similar study, Marybeth Macphee argues the introduction of biomedicine and technology has produced new meanings of health for poorer

Moroccan women. She does not deny these advancements have improved life in some ways; for example, giving birth at a local hospital may be better than giving birth at home alone since a skilled attendant can be present and provide medical assistance if complications arise. However, Macphee writes, "despite advancements in medical delivery . . . women view the process of modernization as having accompanying costs to health" (2004, 375). And in my own research, women often discussed aches and fatigue as results of extra burdens they bear to become the best mothers: the extra trips to the health clinics or the extra cooking and cleaning needed. Whereas these studies are of great value to understanding how cultural change is embodied and how development impacts women's health, Bourqia and Macphee both assume a linear model where development works from the top down, very similar to the INDH. This study destabilizes this assumption by showing development works in the opposite direction as well. Whereas dominant ideologies shape women's practices and beliefs about health, motherhood, and gender, women's interpretations of them also work to inform such rhetoric. Moroccan women ultimately have a great deal of agency and are constantly appropriating practices and ideas for their own purposes while simultaneously navigating multiple discourses.

## THE ISSUE OF LANGUAGE: HINDERING THE BEHAVIORS AND DECISIONS OF THE MODERN BODY

Although Arabic is the official language of Morocco, French is the primary language of healthcare. The written form of Arabic (Modern Standard Arabic) is different from the spoken Moroccan dialect known as *darija*. French was introduced to Morocco when the country became a protectorate. It was implemented as the language of instruction, business, and health services. French officials "aimed at establishing the French language and culture as symbols of 'civilization and advancement'" (Ennaji 2002, 71). After independence, Arabic was rejuvenated and made the official language of the state, and an Arabization policy was launched in the early 1960s to reintroduce Arabic into scientific domains; however, doctors and nurses in Morocco continue to receive their training in French, which causes difficulties in translation and is a hindrance for many working-class women who are unable to read and write. It can possibly prevent them from becoming the responsible citizens and mothers the government wants them to be. Not being able to read their medical charts, prescription bottles, or posters on the walls of the clinics is a barrier within this process and undoubtedly highlights the politicization of language in postindependence Morocco (Boutieri 2012). Moreover, the socioeconomic status of my female participants in and near Rabat plays a key role in the production of this barrier because social and familial structures did not allow many of them to receive a formal education. These various historical and contemporary factors in combination with one another have led to several working-class women not being able to live out their full potential that the INDH guarantees and only works to reinforce the power that medical providers and the government have over women's bodies.

In schools, children begin to learn French at a very young age, and in northern parts of Morocco, Spanish is the second language due to the proximity to Spain. In all of Morocco, French is the primary language of healthcare. This discussion of language is critical to this study given that the health clinics in Rabat where I conducted fieldwork are spaces of multilingualism and (mis-)translation. Women and the medical providers produce new meanings of reproductive practices in this translation process as they grapple to find the right vocabularies to speak to one another (Liu 1995).

The Ministry of Health book that women are expected to purchase, *Le Carnet de Santé de la Femme* (Health Record for Women; *carnet* roughly translates to "notebook" in French) costs a small fee and serves as a record book for women. They are to bring it with them on every doctor's visit because if they see a new doctor, then their records will be in order. It is their responsibility to bring the book. Whereas the main titles of each section are written in Arabic, the actual text of the book is in French. Case in point, family planning appears as *tnzīm al-'usra* in Arabic and *planification familiale* in French at the top of the page, but the tables where the nurse or doctor will record the date of the visit, the method of contraception, and so on, are listed in French only. Clinical staff always wrote this information in French. This leaves women who are unable to read and write Arabic let alone French wondering what the staff has recorded about their bodies and conditions. One woman named Najal, who did not finish high school, looked intensely over her chart as we talked. She pointed to her blood pressure and stated, "This is good I think. I don't know, what is *tension*? I think it is my heart. I'm okay." Najal understood that *tension* or blood pressure dealt with her heart in some way and she was keenly aware of what Fatima was doing when she actually took her blood pressure a few minutes before. But not knowing the precise meaning of the word *tension* led Najal to create a new meaning for it that could change the way she felt about her own body.

Doctors who attend medical school in Morocco receive training in French, which causes numerous translation issues when they attempt to explain procedures or diagnoses to women. In Morocco, as of 2009, 43.9 percent of women above the age of fifteen are able to read and write. This is in comparison to 68.9 percent of men.[30] The female literacy rate in rural areas is estimated at approximately 10 percent.[31] This means the majority of women are unable to understand Modern Standard Arabic and may have very limited knowledge of French. Nadah, the mother of a working-class family I worked with, was unable to read or write. Her first language was *Tachelhit* and she learned Arabic through primary school.[32] She never completed high school. She would ask me how to say household items in French whenever I was at their home. On one occasion she bought a carton of milk at the store and it had gone bad. She handed it to me and explained, "Do you know what's wrong with this? I bought it today, but it's not good. I don't know why. I bought it at the little store, the one right down the street." I looked, the expiration date was written in French and had passed, but Nadah did not recognize this. Cherifa, a young twenty-three-year-old woman who I met at the clinic when she came for a skin rash, asked me to read her prescription bottle because the directions were written in French. She did not understand, and her husband, who worked security, did not speak French well enough to comprehend it either. She said to me in the counseling room, "Can you read this? I don't understand. Look, I tried it but it didn't work. The spots are still there!" After reading the directions and asking Cherifa questions, we discovered that she had not been using the medication properly, which is why it was not working. Doctors and medical staff find it difficult to communicate with patients at times, which strengthens their power and authority over many female patients who seek reproductive and maternal healthcare.

Moroccan women often adopted French vocabularies when they were with the clinical staff, but then would use common words to talk about reproductive practices when they were in the waiting rooms or outside of the clinics. I noticed that the working-class female patients at the three health clinics worked within two vocabularies, rather than the staff making adjustments to their own ways of speaking in order to accommodate the patients. For example, the term for ultrasound in Arabic is *tlfaza*, which literally means "television." Women would commonly use this word when they spoke to each other in the waiting room, but when they would talk to staff they would use the French term *écographie* for ultrasound. In addition, in Moroccan Arabic, the word gynecologist is *ṭbīb al-imra*, which translates as "doctor of a woman." Patients would often say *gynécologue* or *gynéco* for short, which are the French terms for gynecologist. The female patients I observed found unique strategies to bridge this language barrier in order to usurp some control over their bodies back from the medical providers. By suturing this gap, working-class Moroccan women, many of whom did not receive their high school diplomas, also found ways to translate the reproductive practices into terms that made sense for them in order to enhance their well-being, which falls directly in line with the government's outline of responsible citizenship.

## EDUCATION, THE BODY, AND THE FUTURE

Development policies and reproductive health programs in Morocco have kept women's bodies at the center of their interventions, even though their objectives have been expressed in terms of improving well-being and encouraging progress. I have ultimately questioned Morocco's commitment to projects such as the ICPD Action Plan, where women's bodies and reproduction are integrated into the development scheme but yet direct control over them is not the primary goal. I want to conclude with a brief discussion of one of the societal structures that adds to this process of regulation: education. I am not suggesting that the public school system in Morocco is the cause; rather, the government's overall lack of attention to the problems within education has helped reinscribe women and their bodies as "reproducers." Omnia El Shakry notes that at the turn of the twentieth century in Egypt, "mothers came to be responsible for the physical, moral, and intellectual development of children within the nexus of a nascent nationalist discourse" (1998, 126). This occurred at the same time of shifts in discourses surrounding motherhood that focused on "rational upbringing" and the "colonial-hygienic." Dialogues about "good motherhood" concentrated on teaching working-class women the proper techniques of "motherhood along middle-class lines of rational-economic and scientific-hygienic domesticity and childrearing" (ibid., 127). Similarly in Morocco, working-class women expressed their concerns about the education system in that they never completed their high school degrees or they felt that even though they sent their sons and daughters to a public school, they were not receiving a good enough education.

Hayat Diyen sums up the current situation in Morocco concisely, "One of the defects of the old system of education in Morocco is its inability to offer choice and flexibility for students to meet the needs of the modern world . . . Secondary education has to adapt to these exigencies. Secondary education reform in Morocco is, however, full of dilemmas and risks. Facing the reform agenda are immense economic, social and cultural problems" (2004, 211). Upon independence, Morocco adapted the French educational model and incorporated Islamic studies based upon the Qur'an and Arabic as the language of instruction. Structural adjustment programs in the 1980s led to the privatization of education and the development of numerous private Moroccan and international schools.[33] King Mohammed VI once described education in Morocco as a "chronic crisis" (quoted in Tawil 2006, 496). The country is experiencing "multiple symptoms of educational crisis" (ibid.). Between 1990 and 2004, enrollment in primary school increased from 52 percent to 92 percent, and in secondary schools enrollment went from 6 percent to 15 percent. Although there has been an increase in attendance, Morocco has not witnessed positive changes in literacy or unemployment rates and still experiences relatively low enrollments in universities and technical schools. The World Bank has publicly stated that the quality of education in the country is not up to par, especially when compared with other developing regions. It is in need of "urgent reform if it is to tackle unemployment."[34]

Education is key to understanding the creation of modern reproductive subjects for two reasons. The first is it is a key frame through which many of my female participants communicated worry about the future and configured themselves as well as each other as being "good" and responsible mothers. The second is it is one of the main structural factors that reinforces the contradictions found in development policies and the family planning program. The lack of attention to education in all areas including health has produced a greater need to control women's bodies in order to create a national identity built upon ideas of modernity and the need to provide academic and employment opportunities to the next generation. The next chapter explores the education that girls and women receive, both formally and informally, through examining images in reproductive health textbooks, posters on the walls of the health clinics where I conducted fieldwork, and women's and news magazines. Through my analysis, I will show how reproduction and motherhood are being incorporated into the rhetoric of development and how the government and various other organizations, such as the RHO, are framing reproduction and motherhood within the terms of responsible citizenship put forth by the INDH.

# 2 Popular Culture and Textbooks

## Creating Modern Reproductive Subjects and Mothers through Images and Text

The waiting rooms and the counseling rooms of the RHO clinics in Tarma and Zitounia were lined with posters. Some of these posters focused on contraception, while others described good mothering practices. One of the first posters I noticed during my fieldwork was actually located in the adolescent clinic that the RHO runs, located near Tarma. This clinic caters specifically to teenagers and young adults and offers services similar to the one for adults, such as reproductive healthcare, family medicine, dermatology, and psychiatry. The hours are slightly limited to accommodate the school day. Besides the exam room and the counseling room, the adolescent clinic also includes a large room that can be used for gatherings or events, such as those sponsored by its youth club. When I first walked into the waiting room of the clinic, I noticed a poster on the wall above some of the chairs. It is of a woman's hands painted with henna.[1] She is holding a male condom ever so delicately between her index fingers and thumbs.

I took note of this image on several different occasions. What struck me about this poster was the fact that the woman's hands were painted with henna. It demonstrated to me how reproductive technologies are oftentimes intertwined with local contexts as they circulate through different cultures, regions, and even facilities. This image seemed to give the young men and women who visited the clinic the impression that using condoms was an acceptable practice in Morocco. Perhaps it even encouraged them to do so. I found that male condoms were often seen as primarily preventing the spread of diseases, especially HIV, which of course is true. In the public sphere, relatively little attention was given to the fact that they can also prevent unplanned pregnancies. I believe it is for this reason that pictures of condoms were not only found in health clinics, but also seen on billboards and other posters throughout Morocco. The birth control pill and IUD, among other methods of contraception used by women, were not given such positive attention because they cannot stop the transmission of diseases during sexual intercourse. Nevertheless, this poster helped spark my interest in the cultural and medical discourses in Morocco surrounding reproduction and contraception and the different images that have come to be wrapped up within them.

While I was conducting research in Morocco for this project, reproductive health, including family planning, was increasingly gaining attention from the public media, and this attention did not end in 2009 when I returned to the United States nor was it restricted to just Morocco. In 2012, an article in the *New York Times*, titled "New Prime Minister Surprises Moroccans with Support for Abortion," stated that the new minister Benkirane from the PJD is urging the government to relax abortion laws in Morocco in order to counter the estimated high number of illegal and clandestine abortions that take place each year; many of them resulting in the death of the mother. In addition to images in health clinics, articles in popular women's magazines and news outlets in Morocco appeared about contraception, abortion, pregnancy, and motherhood. Some public schools in Rabat offered sexual and reproductive health classes to girls, and the textbooks were saturated with various images of family planning methods, good hygiene practices, the "good" mother, and the modern family. For example, in one of the textbooks immediately before a discussion of contraceptive methods, a cartoonlike image of a family appeared. In it, the mother and father are sitting on a couch and their four children are wreaking havoc around them. All family members are wearing what seems to be old and tattered clothing. The mother is trying to breastfeed her infant while she angrily yells at two of her sons, who are jumping on the coffee table and messing with pictures on the wall. The daughter is clinging to her mother, and the father puts his hands over his ears and has a worrisome look on his face. When students turn the page, they find pictures of different contraceptive methods, including the IUD, birth control pill, diaphragm, spermicides, and male condoms. The book then goes into detail about each of these methods over the next few pages. The very placement of this picture suggests that if girls choose to use contraception to limit and space their children when they are older, then they will not become like this family, who appears not to be well-off financially and seems physically stressed because the parents are unable to control the behaviors of their children. Moreover, textbooks for female literacy classes run by the Moroccan government were also filled with images of what it means to be a "good" mother.

This chapter aims to distill some of the messages promoted by the different images and texts that appeared in the public realm, health clinics, and textbooks in order to provide insight into the discourses in Morocco surrounding motherhood and reproductive health. My intention is that the discourse analysis here will provide a glimpse into the larger social, political, and cultural contexts in which I understood and analyzed my ethnographic data. Philip Rayner, Peter Wall, and Stephen Kruger note, "we as humans experience a need to make sense of the world and the events that take place in it. One important way of doing this is through our consumption of media texts" (2001, 80). Images are key to any analysis of how ideology works. They continue, "On one level, ideology is the system of beliefs that organises the way in which we view the world and the events that take place in it. It follows, therefore, that in our consumption of media texts we will be subjected to the ideological views of the producer of the text" (ibid.). At the level of ideology, meaning appears as natural or commonsense, and because these meanings appear natural, it is difficult for us to always recognize them (Barthes 1972; Eagleton 1991). The suggestion that meanings of images operate on the level of ideology and become like commonsense is useful to my analysis of images surrounding reproduction and motherhood in Morocco. One of the main strategies of Antonio Gramsci's (2000) concept of hegemony is commonsense, making whatever messages seem like the norm or the natural choice. Hegemony or "the process by which a dominant class or group maintains power by making everyone accept their ideology as normal or neutral, through cultural influence rather than force" (Rayner et al. 2004, 85). Consent of the public, or those who are not in power, is then gained through ideology instead of oppression or violence.

For example, take the image I previously described of a woman's hands holding a male condom, which is hanging in the waiting room of the adolescent clinic. Her hands are painted with henna. This is a common practice in Morocco for ceremonies as well as for tourism. Moroccan women will paint the hands and feet of tourists; it is a way for them to earn income and for the tourists to take a souvenir (albeit not permanent) to their home countries.[2] The male condom protects against the transmission of STDs and also prevents pregnancy. It is accessible for many in clinics, health outreach programs, and local shops. I would argue that the henna combined with the condom in this image suggests that the benefits of condom use are recognized in Morocco and that using this method of contraception to protect oneself is a responsible and acceptable practice. If young men or women who enter the clinic accept the "hailing" or "interpellation" (Althusser 1971) of this poster, meaning that they acknowledge they are the addressees and then respond, they are participating in an ideology that constructs them as modern reproductive subjects and responsible citizens. In using a condom during sexual intercourse individuals would be making a thoughtful, calculated, and well-informed decision that would protect them against disease and unplanned pregnancies and ultimately better the nation, which is what this image appears to encourage.

However, the process of consent as proposed by hegemony is not seamless, "Gramsci challenges the ideal that ideology is uncritically accepted by subordinated groups . . . there is a constant state of struggle where dominant ideology is involved in a continual winning and rewinning of the consent of the majority. If a dominant ideology is challenged, it incorporates challenging ideas, thus neutralizing those that threaten its supremacy" (Rayner et al. 2004, 85). In Gramsci's theory of hegemony, the material and social conditions of the targeted (or subordinated) groups sometimes contradict the dominant ideology, which can either cause resistance or alter the ideology. The acceptance of such ideology is not a unidirectional process. Whereas my analysis in this chapter will offer insight as to the cultural and medical discourses surrounding reproduction and motherhood in Morocco, later chapters will illustrate how women have appropriated and interpreted these discourses in ways that make sense for their lives and well-being. Later chapters will also demonstrate how women participate in the ideology promoted by the RHO, state, and development agencies in their own unique ways. I ask that my audience keep in mind my analysis here as they read the remaining parts of the book for this very reason.

## WOMEN'S MAGAZINES: CONSTRUCTING THE AUTONOMOUS INDIVIDUAL AND PERSONAL CHOICE

A prominent theme of recent articles in women's magazines that discussed contraception was individual choice and specifically women's right to choose when to use contraception and which method, but the notion of choice is a highly complicated matter. The ideas promoted by women's magazines sometimes contradicted what I observed in the RHO clinics, where female patients needed to often navigate the advice of the medical staff, the desires of their families, and cultural constructions of womanhood and motherhood. Many articles that I read emphasized well-being and self-improvement through using contraception, but they did not address the dense social and familial networks in which many Moroccan women live. What is striking about these articles is they did not make much, if any, mention of "traditional" methods of contraception that could be used, such as prolonged breastfeeding, the rhythm method, or withdrawal.[3] These articles further complicate the idea of choice by encouraging women to become engaged in the medical realm—another layer of authority in their lives.

Aicha Sakhri, the former editor-in-chief of the popular women's magazine *Femmes du Maroc* (1995–2009), stated that she believes the reason for the success of the magazine is its "'cultural proximity' factor whereby the magazine remains faithful to the Moroccan socio-cultural and religious realities which readers can readily identify" (quoted in Skalli 2006, 82). From my observations, in the attempt to create autonomous citizens, these magazine articles did not particularly account for the varied cultural, economic, and religious discourses surrounding the construction of the individual, but nonetheless they provide an overview to the broader social context in Morocco in which discussions about reproductive healthcare are taking place. In her formulation of contraception as "risk taking," Luker suggests "choices are not always explicit or clearly articulated: in perhaps the majority of life situations, this calculation of the 'risks of life' is a subtle, intuitive, continuing process. This intuitive nature of most of the decision making that goes on in everyday life is sustained by the fact that the social milieu dictates exactly how explicit such decision making can be" (1991, 78). The women's magazines tended to describe reproductive decision making as "explicit" and clear-cut, but drawing inspiration from the work of Luker, I suggest that it is actually anything but when the risks, benefits, and costs are measured against one other.

As I mentioned previously, since I began conducting fieldwork in Rabat, contraception has garnered massive amounts of media attention. A billboard on the road from Rabat to Tarma shows a large photo of a male condom as a way to prevent the spread of HIV. Television programs have been designed around women's health. Women's magazines have run numerous articles on how to prevent pregnancy through the use of modern contraception (like the birth control pill, the IUD, and injections). The popular women's magazine *Famille Actuelle* ran an article in 2008 that outlined various methods of contraception that are currently available to women in Morocco. Just the article's title "Contraception: Choisissez celle qui vous convient" (Contraception: Choose One that Suits You) highlights the ideal that women should be able to choose which method best fits their everyday lives and suits their bodies. The article emphasizes this point especially in the last sentence, "The best contraception is one we choose!"[4] Articles such as this stress that women have the right to choose contraception, and, more importantly, they have a right to take control of their bodies. However, Moroccan women's realities did not always coincide with this rhetoric. The continued desire among men

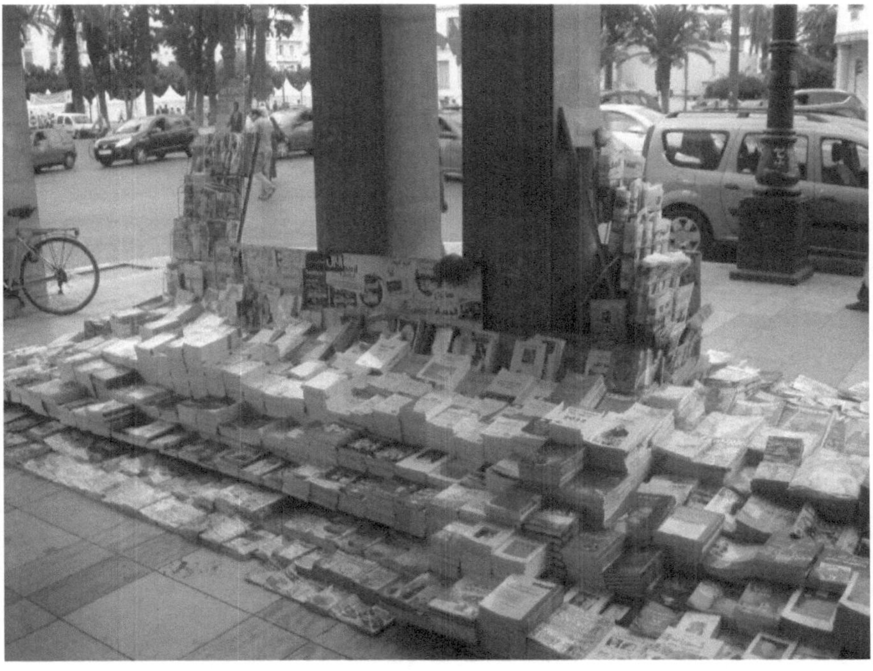

*Figure 2.1* A newsstand with popular magazines and newspapers. (Photo courtesy of Jessica Haney).

and women to have sons along with the existence of patrilocal households produced conflict in patients' lives, with the ideal of personal choice and discourses of reproduction on one side and the sometimes contradictory desires of their husbands or their families on another.

Building on the notion of individual choice is the suggestion found in these magazine articles that contraceptive methods should be adapted to suit women's daily lives. They must choose a method that compliments their lifestyles. In the section *Santé Maman* (Mother's Health) in one popular magazine, a gynecologist in Casablanca discusses how women can easily obtain the birth control pill through pharmacies in Morocco without having to see a doctor first. He states that this is unusual in some countries, but it is acceptable in Morocco and should actually encourage women to use oral contraception. The IUD is more manageable in that it does not require a visit to the pharmacy or doctor for months at a time, but many husbands, according to the doctor, do not look on it favorably. He emphasizes that women have choices when it comes to contraception despite the desires of their husbands. His interview's title, "Every Woman Can Find an Acceptable Method of Contraception" indicates that no matter what the circumstances, all women can find a method to use to limit or space births.[5] The doctor stresses that women should rest assured that they have a broad range of choices since there are diverse methods available to them in the country (*diversité de moyens*). He suggests women should consult a doctor in order to find the best method for them. Although the birth control pill is easily accessible, it might not be the ideal. This interview demonstrates that Moroccan women are expected to accept family planning because not only are methods easy to access, but it is the right and responsible thing to do as citizens. Whereas they have an option of finding the best method for them, using contraception in general comes across as compulsory throughout the article.

"It is essential that women take control of their bodies," said a doctor who is the president of the Moroccan Society for Fertility and Contraception in another popular women's magazine, *Citadine*.[6] In his interview, he emphasized that contraception is not an easy decision, and such choices should be made based on the advice of a gynecologist or other medical professional who has proper training. The doctor encourages Moroccan women to seek out a specialist to discuss their options. Women having control of their bodies and being able to make choices about them is "logical," according to him, because this control will enable them to utilize contraception to avoid unplanned pregnancies. He then links this to the well-being of the nation when he states that contraception is "an excellent thing" because without it, the birthrate will grow, handicapping the country's development. Women exerting control over their bodily practices and lives is not just essential for their health; it is also critical for the entire population of Morocco, according to the doctor. In the articles, both doctors stressed that it is the responsibility of the medical community to inform the Moroccan population about the various methods of contraception available for use, but it is up to women which method they choose. The medical community is to provide women with information and options; however, they need to make the choice to actually use contraception. Women certainly can decide not to use a particular method. They may not use a method due to the plethora of external influences they face, but this is not the "correct" choice they should be making, according to articles like these, which both subtly and overtly link individual contraceptive use to both personal and national gains.

The message behind some of these articles is that there are multiple contraceptive methods available to Moroccan women, which informs the concept of individual choice. Articles detailed many of the methods that women are able to purchase or even receive for free in the public health clinics. In *Citadine*, an article discussed the novel methods of contraception for women, including the hormone patch, the long-term pill that increases the cycle from twenty-one to twenty-eight days, and new versions of the IUD. (Although the IUD discussed in this article, Mirena, was not yet available in Morocco at the time of its publication in October 2008.) [7] In addition, there is great talk of *La Contraception d'Urgence* (emergency contraception) that is to be used after unprotected sexual intercourse or the failure of the primary contraceptive method. In the articles that appeared in women's magazines, there is little discussion of the male condom, even though medical providers stress that it also protects against HIV and the spread of other STDs as well as pregnancy. I realize these articles were published in women's magazines, but this does not mean that women should not be made aware of the benefits of the condom. One of the doctors notes that condoms are the only form of contraception with this double purpose. The lingering question that underlies these articles is: If contraceptive methods are widely available from a variety of sources, then why would Moroccan women choose not to use one, especially because some can be used without the knowledge of men (i.e., the birth control pill)?

Even though these articles from women's magazines were intended to empower women in Morocco and to help them control their own bodies and fertility, notions of the individual and of choice must be qualified and the larger stakes surrounding these constructions must be examined (Sullivan 2001). The heart of the matter is why Moroccan women would not want to use a method of contraception if there are several methods to choose from and they are available for free or at relatively inexpensive prices. Subtle messages promote the normalization of contraceptive use. For example, a second article in a 2008 issue of *Femmes du Maroc* focused on the grave problem of maternal mortality in Morocco. The article stated that reproductive healthcare prior to becoming pregnant and medical care while pregnant is all but free in the public health system. These articles deployed a rhetoric of "easiness" and "attainment," which is in line with the liberal construction of the individual as a "free" and active agent who is responsible for his or her own actions (Rose 1999). At the same time, women are to discipline themselves and each other for not following the mainstream or not making the right choices for their families and society. These magazine articles operated in "moral and material economies" (Andaya 2009, 371) of healthcare where "moral rewards" (ibid., 373)—bettering oneself and the nation through having smaller families by using contraception and regulating fertility—are accompanied by economic gains for the family and the country.

Women were given plenty of choices as to which method to use in order to delay or space their pregnancies in these magazine articles, but they are not given the option to choose not to use contraception, even though they certainly can. Not using contraception is framed as an irresponsible choice by the media. Given the plethora of methods women can choose from in Morocco, they all could find one that is appropriate for them, even those who suffer with a specific physical ailment or those whose husbands would not be pleased with an IUD or a condom. Christa Craven observes in her work on midwives and homebirths, "Medical and state officials have historically justified state regulation and biomedical management of reproductive health care by highlighting the 'pathological' practices of mothers" (2005, 195). I want to point out the notion of privatized, responsible, and modern citizenship promoted by the INDH does not always work to advance women's rights and choices when it comes to reproduction. The rhetoric it promotes also highlights the very complex nature of "choice" for Moroccan women. Sometimes due to social and cultural factors and the medical establishment, women are limited in their abilities to make choices, which calls into question whether modernity really furthers women's agency and control over their bodies and health, as the INDH promises in Morocco. Women's magazine articles frame the choice to not use contraception as a "pathological" practice. This restricted women's choices to fit within the medical community's guidelines and the state's intentions of increasing the quality of reproductive healthcare. At the same time, this also worked to control fertility in order to improve the lives of all citizens—especially those who are young and those who are not yet born.

## FEMALE LITERACY CLASSES: IMAGES OF THE "GOOD" MOTHER

Whereas articles in women's magazines focused on creating an autonomous individual who chooses to use contraception, books used in women's literacy classes centered more on what it means to be a "good" mother. They included images of behaviors and traits that modern mothers should exhibit. The state-sponsored literacy program in Morocco was run with support from USAID. The curriculum of the literacy classes is based on 2004 revisions to the *Moudawana*, some of which included: making the marriage age 18 for both men and women (women's was previously 15), ordering men to see a judge and seek their wife's approval before taking an additional wife, ensuring that both men and women have the right to reside in the household, mandating a written marriage contract, and stating divorce can only take place before a judge and not through verbal repudiation (which was permitted previously for men). The state secretariat in charge of literacy conducted a large-scale survey of twelve thousand households and found that by the end of 2006 illiteracy among Moroccans had decreased. But, approximately 15 percent of children between nine and fourteen years old did not attend school regularly.

The government launched a national program, which sought to teach one million people per year, predominantly women, how to read and write in order to completely eradicate illiteracy by 2015.[8] The curriculum of the government literacy program in part stems from demands of women around Morocco who want to learn more about their rights in marriage and the household. An Amazigh women's activist group stated that it does not matter whether women claim to be Amazigh or Arab, they wanted to learn more about the revisions to the Islamic family code that took place in 2004 and about what they are entitled to within the family unit.[9] The activists argued this is a common goal for a vast majority of Moroccan women despite their ethnic and cultural backgrounds.

Several of the lessons in the literacy classes centered on issues of motherhood and women's familial roles. The lessons detail how the revisions to the code that are to grant women greater rights in marriage, divorce, and the family have impacted practices and constructions of the "good" mother. Here I will not go into great detail about the specifics of the classes, but I will mention every lesson begins with women discussing photos in the textbook. According to Mr. Benjalli, the director of the state-sponsored program, each of these photos deals with one aspect of the *Moudawana* and women are asked to offer their opinions about what each of the photos represents to them in whatever language they feel comfortable speaking (*darija* or an Amazigh dialect). After this, they will learn how to write particular words in Modern Standard Arabic (the written script) that coincide with the photo. Mr. Benjalli explained to me that even though the program has met resistance from some local governments and individuals who he termed "conservatives," the literacy classes have a relatively high rate of success and several women will progress through the various levels and some onto French.

One of the first lessons in the textbook is entitled "The Rights of Children in Identity and Belonging [to the Family]" (*Ḥq al-ṭf'l fī al-huya u al-nsb*). In the picture under the title there is a young woman sitting on a stool, and a little girl is standing beside her. There are two bubbles above the woman's head in the picture that depict her thoughts. In the one, the woman is pregnant. She is looking down, and her hands are crossed over her stomach. Standing next to her is an older man with a beard. He is waving one of his hands in the air. In between the man and woman is what appears to be a wedding ring, but there is a red *X* running through it. In the other bubble the little girl is walking towards a public school, complete with a Moroccan flag on top of the building. Next to the school is a photo of a Moroccan identity certificate. Every child is issued this certificate and eventually will receive a Moroccan national card when they are older. Like the wedding ring, the identity certificate has a large *X* through it. Children cannot attend public school unless they possess this certificate. Prior to 2007, the only way they could receive this document is if their fathers officially recognized them as their children because women could not pass on their Moroccan citizenship to their children until reforms passed that year. In this particular scenario, it seems that the mother did not marry the little girl's father, and therefore the girl cannot obtain the certificate needed to attend school.

The mother has a frustrated and forlorn look on her face as she sits next to her daughter. This picture can be interpreted in several different ways, but one of the messages that may come across to students is becoming pregnant and a mother outside of marriage can be highly detrimental to their children's lives in their future. It could possibly prevent them from receiving an education. Words women learn in this lesson include "my daughter," "lineage," and "strong." Of course, women may not always have a choice in this matter, and the government recognized this in 2007 when it revised the Nationality Code. The new Nationality Code has been deemed a step forward in terms of women's rights in Morocco, but this new regulation also places greater pressure on women to ensure their children are well educated no matter what the circumstances given that they can now pass along Moroccan citizenship to them. This leads to the second message that comes across in the picture: the importance of education. For mothers to be able to pass on citizenship to their children, they are also given the responsibility to guarantee that all of their children receive an education from a formal institution, such as the public school system.

Another lesson in the literacy textbook is called "Responsibility Is Shared in Managing Family Affairs" (*Al-ms'ulya al-mshtrka fī tdbyr sh'un al-'usra*). Under the title there are two images. In both images the same two women are sitting together in what seems to be one of their salons at home. In the top picture, the woman on the right has two thought bubbles above her head. The one bubble shows three women: one is holding a child's hand, another is preparing a meal, and a third is sewing a pink garment. In the other bubble, three men, one of which we presume is the woman's husband, are sitting around a table drinking tea and playing cards. In the bottom picture, the woman on the left has two thought bubbles above her head. The one is of a woman and a child. They are walking together, holding hands. The other is of a man carrying a basket walking alone. In the top picture, the woman holding the child's hand is carrying this basket, but in this picture, the man is. It appears to be filled with vegetables and other goods that he has purchased at the local market. The woman on the left in particular has a forsaken look on her face. It looks as though she is trying to comfort the woman she is speaking with because her husband chooses to play cards instead of helping with household chores. Words that the women will learn how to write in this lesson are: "woman," "door," "teaching/cultivation," "marriage," "man," and "false/untrue."

Something that struck me in these two photos is the fact that the woman is caring for the child in both, even though the man in the bottom picture is taking on other household responsibilities, such as shopping. In both pictures, it is the woman who is watching after the child, although in the second one she has fewer responsibilities because her husband is also helping with the chores. One of the messages that comes across is that even though household duties are to be split up between husband and wife according to revisions of the *Moudawana*, the woman is the one who is to still be the one mainly responsible for the children's welfare. Whereas men may do other chores around the house, women are to ensure that children are reared properly and well taken care of. This not only reinforces the fact that the family is the foundation of Moroccan society, but it also emphasizes that women are to raise the next generation of citizens and nurture qualities that the state considers to be modern, hence the word "teaching/cultivation" in the lesson. Moreover, this message puts pressure on women, particularly those who do not have vast financial means (which are the majority of those enrolled in these courses, according to Mr. Benjalli), to take care of themselves so they can care for their children and to ensure that their children will be prepared to become modern citizens who are productive and will participate in society when they are older.

When I interviewed Mr. Benjalli I asked him what the objective of the program is and why it was created. He responded that being able to read and write allows women to become part of society and gives them greater opportunities for contributing to their households financially. He explained that the lessons center on the fact the familial unit is the foundation of Moroccan society. He said, "The classes talk about the positive aspects of the family. Those are the most important. We do not talk about anything negative like divorce. Then women wouldn't want to be married." Towards the end of our conversation, I inquired as to why women actually enrolled in the literacy classes—what made them want to learn how to read and write? His answer did not follow his response to my first question about the mission of the program. Rather, Mr. Benjalli stated women take the classes to become more knowledgeable about the *Moudawana* and for two other reasons. The first is to better understand health information they receive, such as prescriptions written by the doctors or directions given on medicine bottles. He stressed that women find this to be very important given that they are the ones who primarily take their children to see the doctor. The second most important reason why is because they want to be able to read the Qur'an by themselves and to help their children read and interpret the sacred texts.

These reasons were also expressed to me by Mrs. Sahali, the director of another literacy program in Morocco that focuses on women living in a region of the Mid Atlas Mountains. When I asked her why women in this area would attend literacy classes, she responded they want to educate themselves in order to teach the Qur'an to their children in a manner they feel is appropriate. Like the government-sponsored program, these literacy classes are also based around the revisions to the *Moudawana*. I inquired if Islam was a motivating factor for the women who attend the classes. Mrs. Sahali stated, "Reading the Qur'an is very important for these women. They do not want people telling them the meaning. They want to read it and to teach it to their sons and daughters." She explained being able to read the primary Islamic texts is extremely important for the female students mainly because they can then form their own religious interpretations and opinions and not rely upon the information they receive from other sources, such as television programs, radio broadcasts, husbands, and other family members.

What took me slightly by surprise in my discussions with Mr. Benjalli and Mrs. Sahali was how the women who attend the programs have reinterpreted the purpose of the classes, of being literate, and of the images in the text. Their reasoning for taking the literacy classes differs from what the state and development organization originally intended. On the one hand, the government hopes that women will take on more financial responsibility within the family and society by working outside of the home. To do this, they must become literate. However, working the "double-shift," a common reference in feminist literature, could certainly be more detrimental to women's health and well-being than the state expects (Senturia 1997). On the other hand, women see the literacy classes as helping them enhance their mothering abilities, and this certainly overlaps some of the state and organization's goals. However, they try to improve themselves by being able to read and interpret Islamic texts in order to pass along these specific interpretations to their children and by being able to better understand their families' health needs and the medical terminology used to treat them. So whereas there is overlap between the various objectives of the larger institutions and women themselves, there are simultaneously divergences, which play into how women are creating novel, hybrid notions of what it means to be a "good" mother in Morocco today.

## POSTERS AND BOOKS IN THE CLINICS: TEACHING MOTHERING PRACTICES THROUGH IMAGES AND TEXT

Similar to the images in the literacy textbooks, posters about mothering plaster the walls of the RHO's health clinics. Given a large number of the women I worked with at the clinics were unable to read and write, the visual images these posters provided are of great importance. I often noticed one of the posters about breastfeeding while I was in the waiting room talking with female patients. Fatima explained that these images reinforce what the clinical staff tells women about infant care and childcare. Whereas Fatima is to give impromptu lessons on reproductive health and children's health during the course of the workday, she said that she often becomes too busy to give such informal classes and so she relies on images like this one to do the job for her. This was confirmed to me by another clinic's director, who said she prefers to offer formal sessions in the evenings after the clinic is closed whenever possible because the clinics are too hectic when patients are being seen.

The importance of breastfeeding is emphasized in several of the images that hung on the walls. The images stress breast milk is healthy for babies and will aid their physical development through strengthening their immune systems. In the RHO's clinic in Zitounia, there is a poster in the exam room near the table where the doctor performs ultrasounds. The poster is in black and white and has an outline of a woman breastfeeding. At the top it says "mother's milk" and then goes on to say that breast milk helps protect the infant from illnesses. In the Tarma clinic, a large poster hangs above the chairs that are lined against the one wall of the waiting room. In the bottom right-hand corner is an image of a woman breastfeeding her child. Towards the very top of the poster is a caption in French that reads, "To Succeed at [To achieve] Breastfeeding" (*Réussir l'allaitement maternel*); underneath it twelve steps are listed that women should follow in order to ensure that they will remain healthy while breastfeeding their infants. Many of these steps revolve around mothers' eating habits, such as cutting out sweets and fats from their diets and increasing the number of fruits and vegetables they eat even before giving birth. However, the written instructions are in French, which means that the majority of women who come into the clinic will not be able to read them. They will have to rely on the visual image of the woman breastfeeding and the smaller images associated with some of the steps.

These posters focused on practices that will protect and improve children's health from the moment they are born. I asked both Fatima and Kaoutar how long women should breastfeed their children. They agreed women should breastfeed all of their children for about two years because it is not only important for the baby's development, but it will help them space their pregnancies if they choose to have another child in the future. Prolonged breastfeeding can act as a traditional method of contraception. In addition, they explained Islam advocated prolonged breastfeeding. They referred me to a verse in the Qur'an that recommends children are breastfed for up to two years. The father should support the mother while she is breastfeeding by providing adequate food, shelter, clothing, and all other necessities. Weaning children should only be done if the mother and the father agree upon the timing. The Qur'an reads:

> The mothers shall give suck to their offspring for two whole years, if the father desires to complete the term. But he shall bear the cost of their food and clothing on equitable terms. No soul shall have a burden laid on it greater than it can bear. No mother shall be treated unfairly on account of her child. Nor father on account of his child, an heir shall be chargeable in the same way. If they both decide on weaning, by mutual consent, and after due consultation, there is no blame on them. (2:233)

Whereas breastfeeding was the main theme of these images, another key theme emphasized in posters was having your child vaccinated. In the small public health center in Tarma, every Tuesday, Wednesday, and Thursday there were SME sessions (Maternal and Child Health). Each morning the clinic would offer specific vaccinations for infants and toddlers. The days were divided by age so, for instance, Tuesday was designated for shots given to infants up to six months old and Wednesday was for those between six months and one year. Thursday was typically designated for vaccinations for toddlers. Some days I saw as many as fifty or sixty women line up in the waiting area or in the parking lot of the public health clinic and wait for their children to be vaccinated. All vaccinations at the public health clinic are free of charge. One morning while I was observing an intern directing women and children in the waiting room, I noticed a large poster on the wall. It had a picture of a young boy standing, and above the photo it read in French, "Vaccines are children's rights." This message emphasized that keeping children healthy in part through vaccinations is one of the main responsibilities of parents, particularly mothers. These words stressed that ensuring children's well-being was not optional, but rather a requirement and children's rights. I note here that I say "mothers" rather than "parents" because over the course of my fieldwork, I would estimate that 90 percent of children who were brought to the clinic to be seen by a doctor were accompanied by only their mothers. Their fathers waited in the parking lot or were completely absent altogether. And the photos in the literacy books, even though household chores were to be divided between husbands and wives, still depicted mothers as the ones in charge of children's welfare.

## THE IMPORTANCE OF MOTHERS: TELEVISION PROGRAMS AND ARTICLES ON PARENTING

Television programs and magazine articles on motherhood and parenting methods produced by private companies abounded in Morocco during my fieldwork. When I returned to Morocco in early 2008 for my long-term research, my friend Sarah and her family welcomed me into their home on my first night back in Rabat. A commercial on the television advertised a program that ran on weekday mornings. It featured a woman who had long brown hair and was dressed nicely in a Moroccan *kaftan*.[10] The family members sitting in the living room with me immediately pointed to the television and commented that this ad was for a program directed primarily at women. The program in part discussed how to take care of children. They explained that such programs were very popular in Morocco and that there were several different ones that aired on a regular basis.[11] This particular television program was played at the RHO clinic in Tarma. There was a television, albeit quite old, in the waiting room, and Fatima would often turn it on for the women while they were patiently waiting to see the physician. This specific program featured a woman named Yasmina. She talked about childcare in addition to other household affairs, such as nutritious recipes women could make for their families, decorating tips, and home organization so it would be clutter-free. The women in the waiting room would watch the program intensely, as did my friend Sarah, her mother, and her two sisters.

That same evening, Sarah produced a magazine she had been saving for me. It was *Magella al-Mara al-Arabea: Sītadīn*, the Arabic version of the popular women's magazine *Citadine*. We read the article on breastfeeding together. After flipping through the many pages with photographs of American celebrities like Britney Spears, Sarah came to the section called "My Family, My Children."[12] One of the articles featured was titled "The Last Good Relation between Mother and Child." The article is about how to wean your child off of breast milk and onto the bottle. It emphasized the important bond that breastfeeding creates between mother and child as well as the many health benefits it offers the infant. The article stated that this relationship will end when a child is weaned; however, a new one will begin when the child starts on the bottle. The bond between mother and child will never end. It rather changes as the child develops physically, mentally, and emotionally. What struck me about this article is the stress that is placed upon the emotional and physical bond between mother and child that is created through breastfeeding. Whereas the posters in the clinics pointed out the health benefits of breastfeeding—also important—this article gave greater attention to the attachment between infants and their mothers, which can contribute to their development down the line. A second element of the article that stood out immediately was the photograph that appeared next to the text. It pictured a woman breastfeeding her child. Her wedding ring on her left finger is in clear sight to the readers, which makes a powerful statement as to which women in Morocco are supposed to become mothers: women who are married. Whereas this article and the accompanying image focused on breastfeeding, the statement that such practice creates a lasting bond between mother and child, which changes over time, is part of the larger discourse in Morocco that suggests women are the ones in the family who are primarily responsible for molding and teaching their children and helping them develop in many different ways.

Several other magazine articles focused on the different stages of children's development. One article in *Femmes du Maroc* simply titled "Your Child" (*Votre Enfant*) answers common questions women have about raising children who are still toddlers, those who are pre-adolescence, and those who are teenagers.[13] Under the section on preadolescence, one woman asks what to do about her child who spends the summer glued to the television screen instead of preparing for the next school year or doing outdoor activities. The author of the article states that the television is not an "absolute monster" (*monstre absolu*), but it is important parents actually watch it with their children to understand their desires and sense of humor. It is recommended that parents ask their children to describe the shows they watch and to turn television watching into a learning exercise instead of just a leisure activity. This is actually a very important question as I learned that television is a household staple no matter the social class of the family. It is a crucial media source through which political and social messages can be conveyed, such as through programs about childcare. The last section of the article called "Adolescence" (*ado*) describes what to do when your teenager becomes aloof at home but yet is highly sociable with his or her friends. This can be a concern especially because the family is the foundation of society and its formation is crucial to modernizing the population. The author describes this as a normal part of teenage years and offers questions for the parents to ask in order to uncover their child's unhappiness at home. What this article pointed

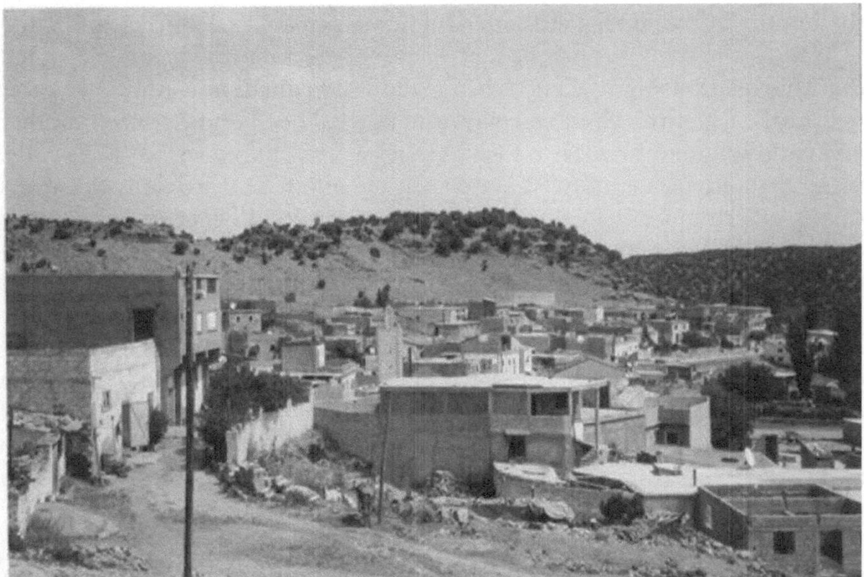

*Figure 2.2* Satellite dishes on tops of homes in a village in Morocco. (Photo by the author).

to is the importance of creating independent and autonomous children who will later become self-governing and productive adults. Children are to be well-rounded through educational experiences (both for academic and personal growth) provided in the home by parents as well as in school.

"Good" mother articles were aimed at women before they give birth and even before they conceive. Several articles discussed prescribed behaviors women should follow when they are pregnant. The magazine *Citadine* published an article in 2009 that details the ideas in society about pregnancy that are true and false.[14] The introductory paragraph states that relatives, friends, and colleagues of pregnant women will sometimes give them contradictory suggestions about what to do while they wait for the birth of their children. It then corrects the false ideas about pregnancy, therefore providing an outline for how pregnant women in Morocco should act in order to have a healthy pregnancy and infant. For instance, one of the last statements the article corrects is that women should satisfy all of their cravings when they are pregnant because if not, their children could have blotches/freckles (*les taches*) on their skin when they are born. The article explains that contrary to this belief, cravings do not have a large influence on the baby and their origins are not specifically known. In general, the prominence of recent articles and television programs about infant care and raising children that are aimed towards women speaks to the importance of mothers in the national agenda of development because of their abilities to influence the physical and mental development of future generations in Morocco.

## CONCLUSION

What are the purposes of women's bodies? How are they to act or be used? What are acceptable and nonacceptable reproductive behaviors for women? What does motherhood mean? The historical moment at which these images and texts were produced is a time of rapid change in Morocco regarding development, gender, and healthcare. New policies and initiatives have brought women's bodies to the center of the creation of the modern nation, and new technologies and practices have made their personal affairs public matters. Their bodies are no longer considered to be on the outskirts of development, as they never truly were, but rather they are recognized to be in the middle of this process. The images that I have analyzed in this chapter certainly pick up on this point as they discuss the importance of women's roles in the family, how mothers should raise their children in Morocco, good parenting practices, and the behaviors and mentalities that children need instilled in them by mothers in order to grow up to be modern neoliberal citizens. Picking up on this point, the next chapter delves into the interventionist practices and spaces of reproductive health clinics and outreach programs and discusses how such practices and spaces aim to create autonomous, self-governing, and self-regulatory citizens as promoted by the INDH and desired by the government.

# 3 Spaces of Intervention
## The Sights and Sounds of Reproductive Health

Dr. Mamouri invited me to his office at the hospital not far from the RHO clinic in Tarma one afternoon for an interview. Even though he was the director of maternity and obstetrics at this public hospital, he also saw patients one day a week at the RHO clinic. I found him to be a well-respected doctor in the local communities. Many women raved to me about the exceptional care they received from Dr. Mamouri, either during routine exams or their deliveries. Dr. Mamouri was extremely knowledgeable and yet very personable. He liked to laugh and was very animated when he spoke. He was born in Morocco and is of Moroccan heritage, but he lived in Belgium for a long time. This is where he completed his medical training before returning to Morocco to practice. During our conversation over tea, he described Morocco as his "mother" and Belgium as his "father." I noticed that more than other doctors he would speak to patients in French instead of *darija*. Each afternoon, after he arrived at the RHO clinic and got himself settled in the exam room, he would poke his head out of the hallway into the waiting room to say "*On y va*" (let's go) to the female patients waiting.

As we chatted in his small office at the hospital, which was located down a busy hallway in the maternity ward, I asked Dr. Mamouri about the differences he found between working at the public hospital and at the RHO clinic in Tarma in terms of structure and the patients he sees at each location. He explained that he enjoyed working at the clinic and actually looked forward to seeing patients there. He was happy at his job at the hospital, but when I asked him why he felt that way, he mentioned that in the RHO clinic in Tarma there is much more organization and the administration is quite good. He motioned with his hands (as if he were chopping something into identical pieces) that things are in order and they are regular. There are rules and guidelines that must be followed by staff as well as patients. For instance, the patients will wait until the counselor or physician calls them, which allows him a greater period of time alone with each patient and also permits him to provide higher-quality care. Dr. Mamouri stated that the hospital seems to lack general oversight in this area and in administration. The RHO clinic is calmer and women do not have to wait as long as they have to at the hospital to be seen by a doctor. Moreover, he appreciates that the proper steps are taken before a woman sees a doctor at the clinic, such as having her vitals taken and recording all the necessary information in her chart. The doctor can then glance at the chart, read over what was written by the counselor, and be better prepared for the visit. He or she knows why the patient has come in that day, her medical history, and what type of services need to be provided. Overall, Dr. Mamouri feels that the system in place in the RHO clinic in Tarma makes for a much more effective and efficient visit than at the public hospital.

In observing the workflow of the RHO clinic in Tarma as well as the one in Zitounia, what struck me time and time again was the great deal of responsibility that is placed on women to ensure that their visits are efficient, the overall clinical processes run smoothly, and they are in good health. From the time women enter the clinic until the time they leave, they are expected to play an active role in their healthcare and their visits. I found this to be true at all stages, whether it is at check-in with a counselor or with the doctor in the exam room. The clinics might be termed Ideological State Apparatuses (ISAs), a concept I borrow from Louis Althusser (1971). Althusser writes of ISAs, "They must not be confused with the (repressive) State apparatus. . . . Repressive suggests that the State Apparatus in question 'functions by violence'—at least ultimately. . . . I shall call Ideological State Apparatuses a certain number of realities which present themselves to the immediate observer in the form of distinct and specialized institutions" (1971, 143). Instead of acting through repression and being located in the public domain, ISAs "'function' massively and predominantly by ideology" (Althusser 1971, 146) and are mainly in the private. Examples that Althusser gives of ISAs include schools, religion, family, legal systems, literature, and the arts. The ideology that governs these apparatuses and is promoted through them is that of the ruling class. Likewise, the rules and guidelines that women and staff must follow in the reproductive health clinics foster the modern mentality that is being promoted through the state, development organizations, and initiatives, including the INDH. Instead of repression, the practices and spaces of the clinics support the development of active and responsible citizens; there is no surprise that this falls directly in line with the type of citizens that the INDH and the Moroccan government seek to create.

In the first volume of *The History of Sexuality* (1990), Foucault addresses the transformation of politics into biopolitics, which he describes as the processes involved in including natural life within the calculations of power. The power over life is no longer aimed to kill, but to invest and to enhance life. It is this investment in human bodies that turns them into objects of knowledge through processes of subjugation. The human body is a space through which power moves discursively and through material practices, such as the childbearing and childrearing practices of the female participants in my research. In *Discipline and Punish*, Foucault writes the management of the body is achieved through "a multiplicity of often minor processes, of different origin and scattered location, which overlap, repeat, or imitate one another" (1995, 138). Foucault and Althusser urge us to look to sites other than the state to understand these minor processes and how bodies become subjugated. This chapter is intended to introduce the audience to the spaces of intervention in which I conducted fieldwork and to the "minor processes" deployed in the medical clinics, such as charting, triage, counseling, and sewing classes, and in the RHO outreach program that aided to the creation of what Foucault terms "docile bodies." How does a policy become embodied? How is the development rhetoric carried out in everyday practice on behalf of the medical providers and patients? What sights and sounds contribute to the creation of the modern reproductive subject and modern citizen in Morocco? I ultimately show it is through these spaces and interventionist practices, which are promoted as empowering and helping women take better care of themselves and their families, that active and responsible citizens who self-regulate their behaviors are created. This chapter provides an overview of the health clinics and the RHO reproductive health outreach program in order to give a sense as to how women come under both the medical and governmental gaze.[1]

## TAKE A NUMBER: ENTERING THE RHO CLINIC AND LEARNING THE SYSTEM

When female patients entered the RHO clinics in Tarma and Zitounia, the first thing they were to do was take a number. The numbers were written on scraps of paper and placed on a chair or small table near the entry. When it was slower, Fatima and Kaoutar would sometimes keep the numbers at their desk. Women would come into the counseling room as soon as they arrived to get one. The counselors would begin calling the numbers one by one for women to come into the counseling room. This was so that women could be afforded privacy while in there and other patients would not overhear why they had come to the clinic that day or their medical histories. As an intern for the RHO, one of my jobs was to take the numbers from the women as they entered the counseling room to ensure that women came in the right order. This was so that the women who arrived first would be seen first by both the counselor and the physician, as the doctor would see them in the same exact order.

Although this system worked the majority of the time, there were times when arguments would break out in the waiting rooms of the clinics over the order in which women would be seen. This was for a few reasons. First, the numbers were written as they would be in French, not Arabic (i.e., 1, 2, 3, 4, 5, etc.). Given that some women who attended the clinic were not able to read or write in French, it was sometimes difficult for them to read the numbers. They would grab any number instead of taking the lowest one available and then become upset when a woman who came in after them would be called by the counselor before they were. Fatima and Kaoutar would often lay the numbers in order on the chair or table, but without a sign instructing women what to do, there was confusion at times. Second, women who were first-time patients to the clinic did not know the system in place for keeping order. They would either just grab a number like the other patients or they would not take a number at all and proceed directly to the counseling room to be seen by Fatima or Kaoutar. This meant they would be going out of order, which upset some of the more seasoned patients who knew the system. In general, Fatima and Kaoutar would explain the system to these women and they would apologize for their mistakes. I noticed that very few became angry because they may need to wait a little bit; most apologized graciously, took a number, and had a seat in the waiting room until it was their turn. And, third, the wait between when women would first enter the clinic and when they would be called by the counselor could sometimes be quite long depending on how busy the clinic was or if Fatima and Kaoutar had meetings in the mornings or inventory to complete. Some women would take a number, leave for a little bit, and then come back. This caused them to miss their numbers being called and would result in an argument either between them and the counselor or between them and the other women waiting when they wanted to reclaim their place in line. I observed that sometimes Fatima and Kaoutar would see them as soon as they returned, whereas at other times they insisted the women take a new number and wait until they were called. The outcome depended upon what services the women wanted and how many other patients needed to be checked in at that time.

Even though the process of taking numbers seems mundane, I saw that women were still expected to regulate themselves and to follow the rules that are in place in the clinics. Fatima and Kaoutar expected that female patients would take the appropriate numbers and wait their turns until they were called. The clinic did not take appointments nor did the staff distribute the numbers to women as they entered. There is an overall system in place to keep order, as Dr. Mamouri mentioned in our interview; however, this system did not work if all of the patients did not participate and keep track of one another. Given there is only one counselor per clinic, Fatima and Kaoutar were too busy working with patients individually in the counseling room to ensure that women took the appropriate numbers when they first entered. Many of the patients returned again and again to the clinics for various services and had to learn the structural system that is in place. When I spent time in the waiting rooms, I saw that women do not particularly learn this system from the counselor, but rather from the other patients also waiting to be seen.

For example, as I sat in the waiting rooms with the female patients, it was evident who were first-time patients at the clinic. These patients would wander in the doorway slowly, looking around for a staff member. They would make their way over to the counseling room, but usually before they could make it there, one or two women would stop them and tell them to take a number by the door and wait to be called. These tended to be the more experienced patients who I had seen at the clinic on several different occasions. Sometimes one of the women would launch into a monologue about how the clinic works, but the majority of the time the new patients would take a number and then be seated until Fatima or Kaoutar called them into the counseling room. On occasion, the new patients would actually inquire about how the clinic worked while in the waiting room and some of the return patients would explain to them the system that was in place.

There was always a buzz in the clinic when Dr. Mamouri or another OB/GYN would arrive for the day. The physicians tended to come in the late morning or early afternoon, after they were finished seeing patients at their full-time place of employment. Things would become a little crazy for a moment, especially if there was more than one specialist in that day, such as the OB/GYN and the dermatologist.[2] Fatima and Kaoutar would need to help the doctors set up, and I noted that they trusted the women would put themselves in order according to their numbers. The chairs in both the RHO waiting rooms lined the walls of the room to form a pseudo-circle. Women would sit in numerical order next to each other, and, as a woman moved into the exam room, they all would shift one seat closer to the exam room door. Fatima and Kaoutar would make a brief announcement that the women needed to sit in the same order in which they were checked in, but then would hustle to the exam room to help the doctor set up his or her things. They rarely helped with the ordering process, unless an argument broke out between patients over their numbers. In general, they left it to the patients to organize themselves and to make sure each was sitting in the correct order and not trying to cut in line.

Female patients were subjects of "responsible communities" (Rose 2000, 1396) within the clinics. Rose notes that under neoliberalism, people are citizens of associations, networks, and social groups. In other words, autonomous individuals are governed not just by themselves but also through communities. As I observed women enter the clinic and take a number, I saw that elements of the INDH and the development agenda in Morocco are being put into action through what seems to be a mundane practice. The system that is in place encourages women to regulate themselves and each other in order to ensure order for everyone in the clinic—both staff and patients alike. It was not the job of Fatima and Kaoutar to govern this process; they left it to the women to do it themselves the vast majority of the time. Women were expected to be responsible and mindful of others, as well as diligent in correcting others, while getting checked in by the counselors and waiting to be seen by the doctor. The development policy in Morocco encourages citizens to develop mentalities of "entrepreneurship" and "participation" through material practices. In taking a number, female patients must exhibit exactly these two traits so that the clinic remains orderly. This allows the counselors and staff to provide higher-quality care to all patients because they will not need to deal with distractions or sort out problems in the waiting rooms while counseling patients or helping the doctors.

## TRIAGE, CHARTING, AND RECORDS: WOMEN'S ACCOUNTABILITY FOR THEIR MEDICAL HISTORIES

After Fatima or Kaoutar called women into the counseling room, the patients would hand over a book to the counselor. These were their record books. Fatima and Kaoutar kept medical charts at the clinics, but these charts were not extremely detailed. They also recorded vitals and all services that were rendered in the women's books. I saw that after the physician would perform a sonogram, a picture was also stapled to a page in the book. There were two different books that women would hand to Fatima or Kaoutar. One was produced by the RHO, and the Ministry of Health made the other, *Le Carnet de Santé de la Femme*. No matter which book the women produced, each one had different sections for education and for charting. The books included discussions of various aspects of sexual and reproductive healthcare and various images of contraception and the female reproductive system. In the back were sections for OB/GYN visits as well as family planning. The counselors would document the date and the service rendered or they would mark the date and type of contraception the woman received at the clinic. The doctor would also make notes in this book during his or her examination and would initial or sign on the line next to the visit's date. During check-in, Fatima and Kaoutar would put the official RHO stamp on the chart as well to denote that the visit took place at one of its clinics.

Women could purchase the RHO book at any of its clinics, and they could purchase the Ministry of Health's book at a public health clinic or hospital. The books ranged in cost between five and ten dirhams (about 55 cents to US$1.12). Fatima and Kaoutar encouraged women to purchase the books if they did not already have one or if the charts in their current book were full. I took note that sometimes women had record books that they carried with them, but they were not one of the ones provided by the RHO or the Ministry of Health. Instead they were plain notebooks that they had purchased from a school supply store or local market. Fatima, Kaoutar, and the physicians at the RHO were fine with this and often suggested that women did not particularly need a formal book from the organization or the Ministry. They just needed some notebook in which their records could be kept.

Books such as these were not just for women's healthcare. When women delivered babies in hospitals, staff encouraged them to purchase a book for their infants that included information about how to care for their newborns and about important immunizations and other medical necessities. These books, titled "Children's Health," also included charts in which staff at the clinics could mark which immunization was given in addition to any other services that the infant received. The book also provides basic instructions on infant and childcare, including nutritional information. There were different books for infants, toddlers, and children. One morning I was able to work with an intern as she saw infants who had come in for immunizations. I observed her write the babies'

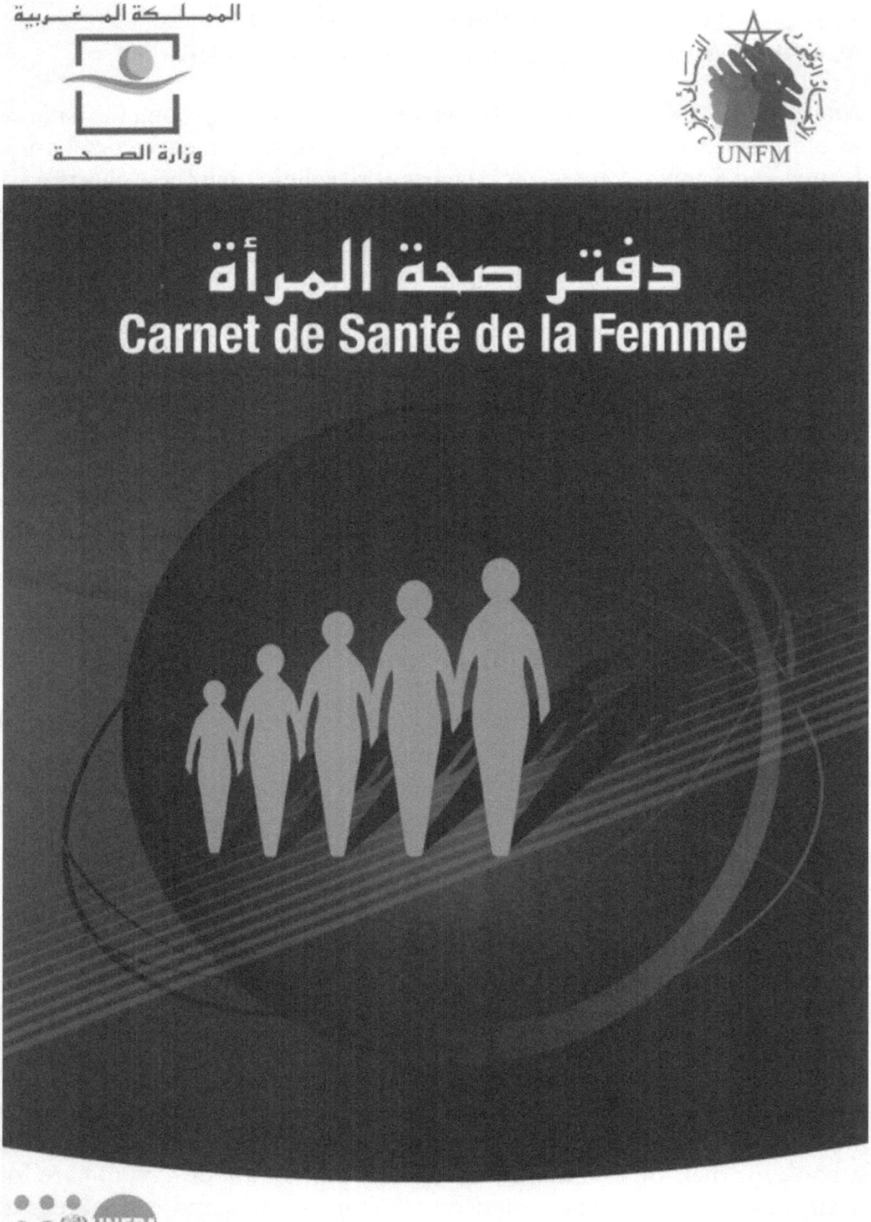


*Figure 3.1* The front cover of *Le Carnet de Santé de la Femme*. (Image courtesy of Ministère de la Santé, Royaume du Maroc).

weights in the books that their mothers would hand to her. After a number of mothers gave her the same book (I noted eight out of eleven mothers on one occasion), I asked what it was exactly and she explained. She went on to state that these books were very important, especially for first-time mothers, so that they can keep their babies healthy. It tells them not only how to care for an infant at home, but also what immunizations need to be administered and when.[3] She said that without these books, some women would never know how important it was for them to take their babies to the doctor especially for immunizations. The children's health book provides the Moroccan government a way to manage and influence women's mothering practices without direct intervention even though it is designed to be purely a self-education tool.

When women did not have books from the RHO or the Ministry when they checked in, Fatima and Kaoutar often asked them if they would like to purchase one. They would explain to them what the book includes and why they should have it: the book includes information about contraception and other reproductive health issues and makes it easier for staff to chart and keep track of the services provided. If the patient hesitated about the cost, the counselors would suggest they purchase a plain notebook instead, which might be cheaper. I asked Fatima why women needed books at all. I knew that the charts in the clinics were relatively less detailed than the records kept in the books, but I was curious why she thought they were a necessity for care. She stated that because some women live far away from the clinic, they would see other doctors or medical personnel at other facilities. If the women would consistently have all the doctors or staff they see chart in their books, then it would be much easier to keep track of what services they had already received, where they were provided, and who provided them. This can cut down on women having duplicate services or unnecessary procedures and allows them to have a more complete medical record. This in particular made it much easier for the physician to diagnose and treat patients.

I showed the book from the Ministry of Health to Mr. Benjalli, the director of the national literacy program, one afternoon when we met for coffee. The program uses health information in its classes and teaches women Arabic words they would see and use at a clinic. What angered the director about the book is that the charts are predominantly written in French and not Arabic given that the language of healthcare in Morocco remains to be French. Physicians are often trained in French in Moroccan medical schools and so are nurses and other medical staff. Oftentimes I observed the staff at the RHO and public health clinic would chart in French, which would leave women who were illiterate or learning how to read and write left to wonder what they were recording about their visits and bodies. Mr. Benjalli was pleased that the books existed and that women can receive better medical care because of them, but at the same time he was disappointed because the books still stripped some women of power over their medical decisions and bodies because they could not understand what was being written in the charts unless they continued their literacy studies.[4]

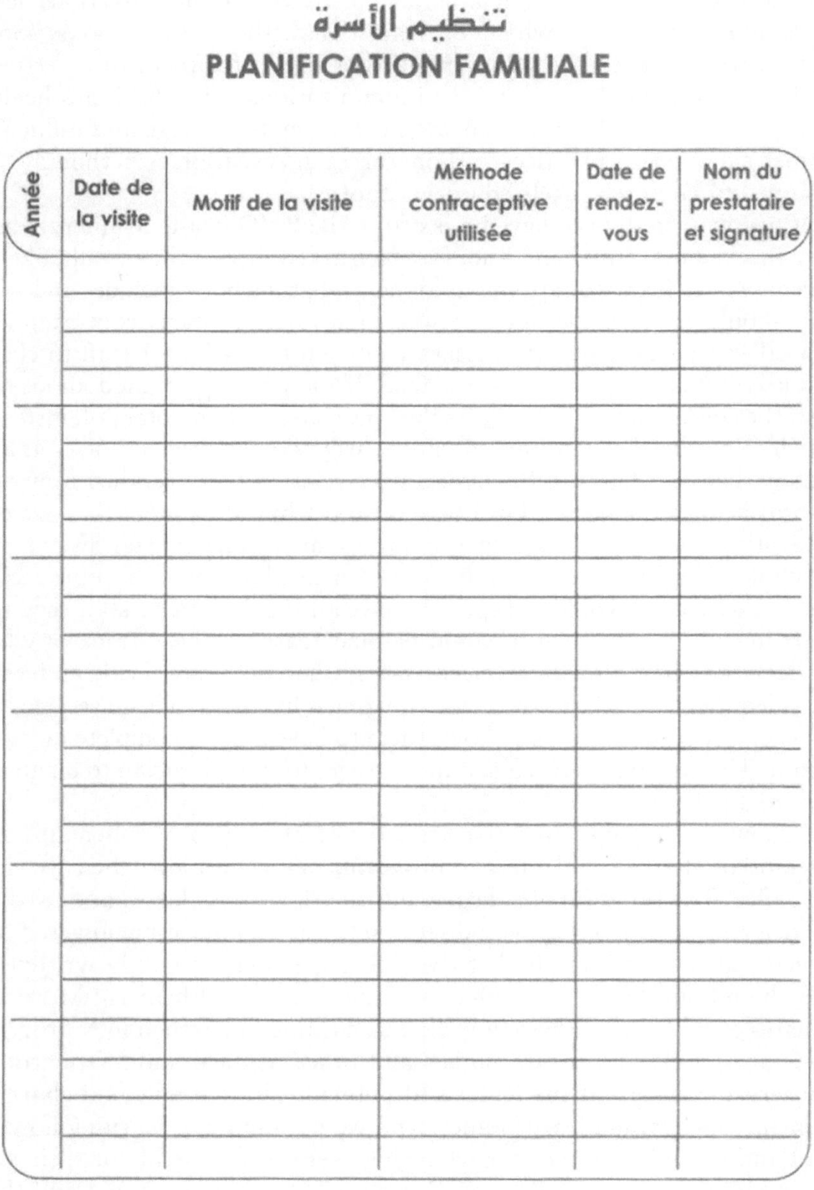

تنظيم الأسرة

**PLANIFICATION FAMILIALE**

| Année | Date de la visite | Motif de la visite | Méthode contraceptive utilisée | Date de rendez-vous | Nom du prestataire et signature |
|---|---|---|---|---|---|
| | | | | | |
| | | | | | |
| | | | | | |
| | | | | | |
| | | | | | |
| | | | | | |
| | | | | | |
| | | | | | |
| | | | | | |
| | | | | | |
| | | | | | |
| | | | | | |
| | | | | | |
| | | | | | |
| | | | | | |
| | | | | | |
| | | | | | |
| | | | | | |
| | | | | | |
| | | | | | |
| | | | | | |
| | | | | | |
| | | | | | |
| | | | | | |

*Figure 3.2* The chart for family planning in *Le Carnet de Santé de la Femme*. (Image courtesy of Ministère de la Santé, Royaume du Maroc).

What struck me about these educational and record books produced by the RHO and the Ministry of Health is that they required women to be active participants in their own medical care. Female patients needed to make sure that they brought the book with them each time they saw a doctor and that the medical staff completed their charts. Women were the ones primarily responsible for their medical records, not particularly the staff at the RHO clinics or the public health clinic. If they forgot their books, this did not mean that they could not receive care, but both Fatima and Kaoutar would remind women how important it is that they have a complete (or as complete as possible) medical record for the physician. By having this record, the doctor could see what services had been rendered in the past, what medications they were prescribed, and what medical conditions they suffer from, all of which would expedite the treatment and diagnosis of their patients. In this discussion of the books, what I want to emphasize is that women were being granted a great amount of responsibility for their medical services as well as for taking care of their bodies and overall health. This practice not only facilitated care within the clinics, but it also made women accountable for their charts and records. I would like to point out that one of the main tenets of the INDH and development agenda in Morocco is to hold citizens accountable for their decisions and behaviors; similarly, women were being held accountable for their medical histories and expected to actively participate in their completion by bringing their books to every doctor's visit. The books not only made it easier for the counselors, nurses, and doctors to treat their patients, but they also encouraged women to take part in their own healthcare and ultimately bettering their bodies and well-being.

## FAMILY PLANNING COUNSELING SESSIONS: TO ACCEPT OR NOT ACCEPT CONTRACEPTION

The books produced by the RHO and Ministry of Health had a separate section in which the medical staff charted women's use of family planning. Staff members mark when patients received contraception and what type. Whereas women in Morocco, especially married women, are given several different methods of contraception to choose from, such technology can still be used to implement social controls over women's reproductive behaviors and to create the modern citizens that the state intends. Reproductive technologies are seen as advancing women's agency and simultaneously as "threatening to individual rights" (Nelkin 1995, 449).

Female patients of the RHO clinics who give birth in a hospital are to return shortly after for a checkup. At this visit, Fatima and Kaoutar reiterated to me that the staff is not allowed to force women to accept any method of contraception. Women must accept a method on their own and are allowed to choose which one is best for them. However, I saw that within the clinical setting, women's choices are limited to those that are considered beneficial to themselves and their families. This framing does advance women's agency, but at the same time it is an attempt to produce self-regulating and responsible citizens who make well-thought-out choices about their lives. At home, women can easily choose not to use contraception, such as not continuing to take the pill, but my focus in this section is to show how the promotion of this reproductive technology aids to the construction of modern, responsible, and active citizens.

After a woman gives birth, she is instructed to return to the RHO clinic in approximately three months for a consultation with the doctor. The time period in between birth and consultation is slightly longer for a woman who has had a cesarean section (C-section). Fatima explained that when she would counsel a woman who had returned to the clinic after having a baby, she would give the woman three options: "I tell her that she can use the same method that she was using before she became pregnant, she can choose to change methods if she wants, or she can begin to use a method if she was not before." She continued, "Women should not become pregnant again so soon. They need to use contraception. We have contraception that will not be a problem if they are breastfeeding." The RHO even carries pills with very low doses of hormones so that they are safe for mothers who are still nursing and want extra protection against pregnancy. In general, Kaoutar agreed with Fatima's statement, but she also confirmed that several women attend the clinic for various reasons over extended periods of time, so coming in after they give birth for an annual exam or consultation is not uncommon. What is striking in their explanations is choosing not to use contraception is not an option inside of the clinic; this is not to say that women who chose oral contraception could not throw the pills away or not take them once they returned home. However, in this space of intervention, using contraception was the only suitable choice. Fatima and Kaoutar were clear that women can choose the method, but they were not allowed to leave the clinic without receiving contraception. Although women were given leeway as to which contraceptive method they chose at the RHO clinics, there was little room for them to work around the medical recommendations of the counselors.

Contraception was not only integrated into post-birth consultations but also into routine doctor's visits as well at the RHO. In the main exams of the Tarma and Zitounia clinics there was a sheet of paper hanging near the medicine cabinet, where supplies were kept for ultrasounds and other basic procedures. On this sheet were directions for OB/GYNs and general practitioners. At the top of the list for family physicians, it stated they should incorporate discussions of contraception into their conversations with female patients during their examinations. According to the sheet, it did not matter the reasons why female patients had come to see them; they must make an effort to talk to these women about family planning regardless. The generalist I worked with, Dr. Kinjalli, who also worked at a public health clinic in Tarma several days a week, confirmed she would discuss contraception and pregnancy with the majority of female patients who came to see her even for common ailments. This did not include women who were going through menopause, who were pregnant, or women trying to become pregnant. Dr. Kinjalli recommended contraception for women based on their health needs, performed gynecological consultations, and did follow-ups on the placement of women's IUDs, but if there was an issue she was unfamiliar with or felt uncomfortable treating, she would refer patients to one of the OB/GYNs at the clinic for further treatment.

On the list for OB/GYNs, it reminded them to ask female patients if they are currently using a method of contraception at the beginning of each consultation. But again, this does not apply to women who are pregnant, attempting to conceive, or have gone through menopause. However, the sheet did not specify women's marital status; they were instructed to speak to all women whether they were single or married. Dr. Senah stated she would always ask women who come in for the first time or for their annual exams if they were using contraception. She stated to me in between patients, "I will always ask if they are using a method. If they aren't and don't want children, then I tell them to see Fatima when they leave for contraception. I talk to them about the methods." Overall, doctors and counselors at the RHO clinics do not give women the choice of not using contraception unless they are trying to become pregnant. Ultimately, although affording women some control over their bodies given they can select a method, this also reduces the amount of control that they have because there is only one ultimate decision that can be made: to accept family planning.

The counselors at the RHO clinics will sometimes make home visits to women in the local area as a way to check up on them after they give birth or to see those who have not returned to the clinic for care. This is also a way for the counselors to talk to other men and women about the services the clinic offers. Rahma, the director of annother RHO clinic located in a poorer quarter of Rabat, explained that staff will often travel to the shantytown across the street from the clinic to distribute methods of contraception and to provide men and women information about reproductive healthcare. Rahma pointed out the exam room window and said to me, "Look over there, you see that *bidonville*? It is such a shame. We go there. We tell them about contraception and how to keep their children healthy. Many of them do not go to school. They are very poor. We try to help."

In her work on motherhood in Greece, Heather Paxson argues that the state and health workers in the country advocate modern models of womanhood, which include attention to reproductive health and the promotion of women's autonomy, but they "ultimately compound their reproductive accountability" (2004, 36). She finds that these modern models do not particularly give women more choice or agency but actually limit them in many ways. Similarly, in my observations of family planning counseling sessions in Morocco, I noticed that whether it was with a counselor or a doctor, women were directed along one path—the path to accepting family planning—but were allowed to make different decisions along the way as to the process itself. They could choose which method to use according to what would best suit their lives and needs. The counseling sessions and practice of incorporating contraception into all visits granted women a degree of agency and personal choice, but their overall structure still worked to create modern citizens who make certain responsible choices about their bodies.

Reproductive choices in Morocco are extremely intricate, and citizens must negotiate several structural and cultural forces in their decision making. I found that contraception is framed by the medical professionals I observed more so as a way to produce healthy children and families than as a method to limit births. The ultimate "benefits" were emphasized and power was invested in life (Agamben 1998). Moroccan women's choices were not particularly expanded with the introduction of contraception, even though the national development policy promises to increase the number of choices citizens have as a means to improve their lives. Greenhalgh (1994), in her work on family planning and the one-child policy in China, contends most women are viewed as "victims" of family planning and policies, but when we take a closer look, it is revealed that they are also active "agents" in the practice. The female patients at the RHO and public health clinics often did use contraception to optimize their lives and to better their health, yet their choices were actually hindered in the clinical setting due to the need to produce responsible citizens who always make the best decisions when it comes to their lives. This means that choosing not to use contraception is then taken completely out of the equation.

## VOLUNTEERS AND THE RHO COMMUNITY OUTREACH PROGRAM

In addition to the health clinics the RHO runs throughout Morocco, the organization also runs six community outreach programs. Each mobile unit focuses on providing contraception (birth control pills and male condoms) and information about sexual and reproductive health to rural areas and smaller towns. The outreach teams are based in six major cities in Morocco (Casablanca, Rabat, Fes, Marrakech, Tangier, and Agadir) and will travel to neighboring areas. Amin, a man in his late forties, was in charge of the outreach program in Rabat. He had worked with the RHO for a number of years in a variety of capacities. He not only was in charge of the outreach program for the region, but would also run errands for the office staff at the headquarters and deliver supplies to different RHO clinics in and near Rabat. Amin allowed me to travel with him on several occasions to the more rural areas of the Rabat region, where he would deliver contraception and pamphlets on the sexual and reproductive health services the RHO offers in its clinics.

Whereas counselors at the RHO would make home visits from time to time, the mobile units were crucial to its mission of offering everyone, regardless of age, marital status, or location, high-quality and low-cost sexual and reproductive healthcare. The RHO recruited members of the communities to be its volunteers. They would be paid a small fee for their work. I asked one of the executive staff members at the RHO how they would select the volunteers. She explained that they would first meet with local officials or well-respected members of the community to discuss the possibility of establishing an outreach program in the local area. Once the RHO received permission, they would request names of people who would make good volunteers or places they could go to recruit individuals for these positions.

I found that the volunteers ranged in occupation and status in the community. In some of the smaller towns that Amin and I would visit, the volunteers worked for small community health centers that were privately run. One of the workers at one of these facilities actually lived in the clinic so he could see patients nearly twenty-four hours a day. He had a small kitchen and bedroom set up right off of the exam room. These small health clinics in the rural areas did not offer contraception, so workers would pair with the RHO in order for patients to be able to receive birth control pills or male condoms at a low cost. Other volunteers were regular members of the community, such as the twenty-six-year-old clothing store owner I discussed in Chapter 1 or a middle-aged woman who owned a small corner store that sold basic grocery items, snacks, and drinks.

Whereas some volunteers had medical training, others did not. The RHO volunteers did not have to have a medical background. They received basic training from the organization each year so they could address questions about sexual and reproductive health, or at least point people to a source where they could find the answers. The volunteers were expected to visit people's homes to distribute information about the organization and sexual and reproductive health in general and to teach them how to properly use the contraception they could provide. The volunteers' homes or shops would receive a seal from the RHO that could be placed on or near the front door so that the community knew where birth control pills and male condoms could be purchased. When I asked one volunteer what made the program so attractive to individuals living in his community, he said it was the cost and the fact that anyone could purchase them despite age or marital status.

Amin had a set schedule when he would visit each of the areas serviced by the Rabat mobile unit. All of the volunteers knew which days he would be delivering supplies. The volunteers would sell the condoms and birth control pills to individuals in the local community and then when they would run out, they would take orders for Amin. When he arrived, the volunteers would pay one dirham (US$0.10) for each condom and three dirhams for each supply of birth control pills (US$0.33). They would then sell the products for an additional dirham each, which they would then keep for their time and effort. The volunteers were able to make some money through this position but certainly not enough to live on. Sometimes the volunteers said they would collect the money ahead of time so that they were not left with lots of supplies to sell, but most of the time they would just take the order and the customers would pay when they received the contraception. Nearly all of the volunteers would buy extras to have for new customers or those who did not put their orders in on time. The volunteers acted as the middlemen between the RHO and the local communities. Instead of Amin traveling into the communities to deliver the supplies and information directly to individuals, the RHO empowered members to do this instead. This not only made the program a success, according to the staff members at the RHO headquarters, but it also made Amin's trips, and those of other outreach coordinators in Morocco, much more effective and efficient.

I was interested in learning why the executive staff at the RHO believed that having community volunteers made the outreach program popular and successful. When I asked Noor, the former director of programs at the RHO, why this was, she explained that it helped if community members were the ones distributing the information and contraception, not staff members from the RHO. She said it made people feel more comfortable if they approached their neighbors or local shopkeepers for contraception rather than a stranger because they may be more familiar with them. Also, if they saw other community members, such as their neighbor or a relative, approaching the volunteers for supplies, it was much easier for others to purchase supplies, too. Noor believed the outreach program was a win-win situation. Amin could cut down on the amount of time he spent in each community, which meant he could visit more places in less time, and local individuals could receive supplies from people that they trusted and were more comfortable being around. According to Noor, this is also why the RHO recruited both male and female volunteers. If people felt more comfortable buying contraception from a same-sex volunteer (or an opposite-sex volunteer), then they had the opportunity to do so. The goal of the RHO outreach program was to make obtaining contraception as easy as possible for everyone and to create an atmosphere in the rural areas that was accepting of family planning. If well-respected community members endorsed the outreach program, then the RHO hoped more individuals in the local areas would join either as volunteers or as participants.

In a sense, the RHO had stepped out of the rural areas in terms of providing reproductive healthcare and instead placed the responsibility upon the community itself to provide for its members. The RHO has not built clinics in these small towns and rural communities, but rather provides members the supplies and tools needed to ensure that individuals are aware of and use contraception. Drawing on the social science literature, it can be argued that the outreach program is an additional form of surveillance over people's reproductive decisions and practices given that community members (as well as the state and development agency) are mainly responsible for producing particular reproductive subjects who regulate their reproduction (Foucault 1995; Greenhalgh 1994; Kligman 1998). It is anticipated that individuals will purchase contraception from the volunteers and use it regularly once they know their friends and family members also buy supplies; therefore, they will begin to regulate their own behaviors. However, scholarship in public health shows that community-based medical programs and those that incorporate local volunteers have a higher success rate at getting more people to accept family planning or to receive proper medical care (Pence et al. 2007; Phillips et al. 1999). The RHO sees its outreach programs in Morocco as empowering members of local communities, particularly the volunteers, to take care of their own bodies and lives and to help others take care of theirs. Rather than the RHO staff, it is the program volunteers who work to produce "morally responsible individual[s]" (O'Malley 1996, 194) within their own communities who make life choices that will enhance their well-being, overall health, and their families' lives. Because many of the rural areas where the RHO has an outreach program in place were not well-off economically due to relatively high rates of unemployment, community volunteers were also to emphasize the financial benefits of having fewer children or spacing births properly to all individuals they encountered through their program.

## SEWING CLASSES AT THE RHO HEALTH CLINIC IN TARMA: AN ADDED BONUS

The RHO health clinic in Tarma offers sewing classes to all of its female patients and their families or friends. All women can participate in these free classes instructed by two teachers, Nora and Haneez.[5] Even if women already know how to sew well, the RHO provides them with a space in which they can socialize and work together. Nora and Haneez would teach those who did not know how to sew or would have liked to improve their skills for free of charge. In addition, they guided those who were more experienced in their projects. All of the participants in the sewing classes were extremely talented and made pieces of clothing in addition to home décor and items for special ceremonies and celebrations, such as weddings.

Several of the women who participated in the sewing classes were patients at the Tarma clinic, but they also came to sew on the days that they did not have appointments with the doctor. Each morning when I arrived at the clinic, there would be anywhere from three to ten women in the sewing room with Nora and Haneez. They would sew during the mornings until the clinic's staff, including the teachers, took a lunch break. The teachers would return in the afternoon for a few additional hours and open the room again for women to work. In general, the women in the classes knew each other well, and most of the ones I spoke with had been participating for an extended period of time. When I asked Noor why the organization offered the sewing classes, she responded that like dermatology or family medicine, it is an added service intended to keep female patients attending the clinic and to attract new patients. If patients attend the classes on a regular basis, Noor believed that they would be more likely to seek additional services at the clinic. In other words, the sewing class is a way to get women through the clinic's door and to encourage them to use its medical services while they are there. I noticed that Nora and Haneez would often remind women during the classes how important it was to talk with Fatima about family planning or other medical concerns and to see the doctor when necessary.

Whereas attracting new patients and encouraging women to use additional services at the clinic were two main objectives of the sewing classes, sewing was also promoted as a way for women to contribute economically to their families and to help their families improve their financial standing. When I asked women what they did with the items that they produced in the class, many of them said that they would sell them for additional income. Nora said to me that many of the female participants come from the local area, and the clinic is located in a working-class community. The vast majority of the women in the classes do not come from money and their families do not have a great deal of financial resources, so selling the items that they produce is a way for them to help, too. In addition, she said that sewing is flexible and can be done at home as well as in the classroom in case the women have small children to take care of during the day. Nora and Haneez described sewing as a relatively simple way for women to bring some extra income into their households given that many of them do not hold regular employment outside of the home.

Colin Gordon writes that the "real basis of the state's wealth and power lies in its population, in the strength and productivity of all and each" (1991, 10). In order for profitable accumulation to occur and the market to develop, people's bodies and minds must be managed accordingly (Burchell 1996). One goal of the INDH is to increase individuals' income-generating activities so that segments of the population can bring themselves out of their poorer financial standing in society. Once they accumulate wealth, they will have a broader range of choices and will be able to make better decisions about their lives. Both of these end results are expected to impact the nation in positive ways—the poverty rate will decrease and Morocco can become a competitor on the global economic stage. However, in order for this to occur, individuals must be given the education and the tools needed in order to help bring themselves out of poorer economic circumstances, such as technical skills like sewing. Once citizens receive these, they are expected to use them to their full advantage. Zemni and Bogaert write of the INDH:

> The rationality that comes forth with the [INDH] endeavours to combine a 'mix' a responsible, moral individual with the economic rational and calculating individual.[6] "Bringing" the excluded back in the "realm" of virtuous citizenship therefore seems one of major challenges. What is described as the "modern way of engaging these problems" is in fact politics that reduce social and economic structural problems to questions of personal or individual responsibility. (2009, 102)

I suggest that the sewing classes are a way for working-class women from the local communities in Tarma to become part of the "'realm' of virtuous citizenship" in Morocco. The classes are a tool that the RHO provides women so that they can earn money to help themselves, their children, and their families. As Zemni and Bogaert observe in their project, larger economic issues in Morocco are being reduced to notions of personal responsibility. The RHO staff and the sewing teachers talk about the classes as helping women contribute to their household's finances, improving their children's well-being and education through additional income, and making them feel better about themselves and their own lives. I argue that sewing is not just a technical skill that women learn at the RHO clinic in Tarma, and it is more than just a way to keep patients coming to the clinic. It is also a means for women to become entrepreneurial and competitive, to make calculated choices, and to become responsible Moroccan citizens who use the tools provided to them to help improve their economic status.

## CONCLUSION

Whereas the first two chapters of this ethnography gave a broad overview of the current development initiatives and images surrounding reproduction and motherhood in Morocco, this chapter has taken a deeper look at the practices and spaces of reproductive health. It sets the stage for the following three chapters of this book. My objective here has been to illustrate how different practices in the health clinics and of reproductive health more generally, such as the RHO community outreach program, actively contribute to the creation of modern citizens and modern reproductive subjects in Morocco. The spaces and practices of intervention mold women into the types of citizens that the INDH and the government's development agenda consider to be modern—responsible, self-governing, calculating, and willing to take advantage of information and services that will improve their lives and bodies. The second part of this book will build upon this chapter in that it shows how women actually appropriate these practices of intervention to create new identities, understandings of Islam, and novel ideas of womanhood and motherhood. My upcoming analysis will demonstrate that Moroccan women tend to fashion these practices in ways that were unintended by the government, RHO, and development agencies, but that nonetheless still fit within the development rubric of responsibility and active participation.

# Part II

# 4 Contraception and Living a Quality Islamic Life

There is little doubt that headlines of recent news articles such as "Nearly 1 in 4 People Worldwide Is Muslim" (Greene 2009) and "Let's Admit It: Honor Killing in the West Is by Muslims" (Chesler 2012) can raise the public's anxiety about the global Muslim population. Further uneasiness about this burgeoning population comes about in the opening sentence of the first article published on the CNN website, "Nearly one in four people worldwide is Muslim—and they are not necessarily where you might think" (Greene 2009). This opening statement suggests that the Muslim population is not confined to the "heartland of Islam," (Eickelman 2002) the Middle East. After the tragic events of September 11, 2001, migration of Muslims raises concern about the potential for terrorist acts by Muslim fundamentalist groups who have settled in the West, in places like the United States, Canada, or Europe. Jennifer Johnson-Hanks writes, "From scholarly books to newspaper articles to mass culture sources, it seems fair to surmise that Muslim fertility has come to matter politically in the United States. People write about it, believe it to be excessive, and fear it" (2006a, 13). These types of news headlines reiterate Johnson-Hanks's point about the political nature of Muslim fertility. Muslims' reproduction and, more importantly, their bodies have become the subjects of political and popular scrutiny in part to prevent the international threat of violence by future generations.

In the best-selling book *The Clash of Civilizations and the Remaking of World Order*, Samuel Huntington suggests that high fertility rates among Muslims is one of the main causes of "Muslim militancy, militarism, and migration" (1996, 121, cited in Johnson-Hanks 2006a, 13). Huntington argues that "Muslim population growth has generated large number of unemployed and disaffected young people who became recruits to Islamist causes, exert pressure on neighboring societies, and migrate to the West" (1996, 211, cited in Johnson-Hanks 2006a, 13). Huntington is not the only author warning his audience of the potential dangers of Muslim fertility rates. In a 2010 article that appeared in *Foreign Affairs*, Jack Goldstone (a current professor of public policy) highlights the potential threat posed by Muslim youth if states or foreign governments do not control the population. He argues that improving the relations between Muslim majority countries and countries in the West (i.e., the United States and Europe) is a critical move due to the "growing demographic weight of poor Muslim countries and the attendant increase in Muslim immigration" (2010, 37). Goldstone writes of Muslim youth:

> Their populations are continuing to grow and indeed are expected to increase by 475 million between now and 2050—during which time, by comparison, the six most populous developed countries are projected to gain only 44 million inhabitants. Worldwide of the 48 fastest-growing countries today—those with annual population growth of two percent or more—28 are majority Muslim or have Muslim minorities of 33 percent or more. It is therefore imperative to improve relations between Muslim and Western Societies. This will be difficult given that many Muslims live in poor communities vulnerable to radical appeals and many see the West as antagonistic and militaristic. (Ibid.)

The underlying concern of Huntington's book and Goldstone's article is that there is an increased threat of violence due to the migration to the West of poor Muslims who are engaged with fundamental Islamic organizations. This migration results from a lack of education and job opportunities due to corruption in the public and private sectors in their home countries and the fact that there are not enough resources to increase the number and quality of job openings and educational institutions for Muslim youth. The solution is then to make the control of Muslim fertility a worldwide priority in order to prevent the movement of Muslims from their home countries to the West and to thwart future terrorist acts by members of Islamic groups who promote the use of violence against non-Muslims and each other.[1]

Anxiety surrounds Muslim fertility in popular and scholarly discourses. Articles like Goldstone's, titled "The New Population Bomb: The Four Megatrends That Will Change the World" (2009), contribute to the general public's panic over the increasing Muslim population worldwide. It is true that roughly one in four people in the world is Muslim, but one in five Muslims actually live in countries where Muslims are a minority (Greene 2009). Overall, there are approximately 1.57 billion Muslims around the globe, according to the Pew Forum on Religion and Public Life (Pew Research Center 2009), which represents 23 percent of world's population of 6.8 billion. The MENA is home to only about one in five of the world's Muslims, "making up a smaller and smaller percentage of the worldwide Muslim community" (Reza Aslan, quoted in Greene 2009). In the United States, the Muslim population "is an estimate and somewhat controversial depending on which communities are included. But it is generally accepted that there are between 3 and 5 million Muslims in the country, and that this number is growing" (Ibrahim 2012). Whereas the Muslim population continues to grow outside of the "heartland," in reality the fertility rates in several MENA countries have declined in recent decades and continue to decline dramatically.

Eight of the fifteen countries in the world that have experienced the biggest decreases in fertility rates since 1980 are in the MENA. This list is led by Iran, followed by Tunisia, Algeria, the United Arab Emirates (UAE), Libya, Kuwait, Qatar, and Morocco. Hania Zlotnik, the director of the population division at the United Nations Department of Economic and Social Affairs since February of 2005,[2] congratulated governments in the Islamic world for helping facilitate a drastic drop in population growth. She credited education and access to family planning even in "conservative Muslims states" as playing a large role (Macfarquhar 2009). Zlotnik is quoted in the *New York Times* as saying at a population conference, "In most of the Islamic world, it's amazing the decline in fertility that has happened." She continued, "Even in cultures that are Muslim advances of very big quantity can be made, if the government has enough commitment to provide services and the social infrastructure that validates those changes" (quoted in Macfarquhar 2009). High fertility rates are now an exception rather than the norm in the Muslim world, with only Yemen falling into this category. Zlotnik suggests that those countries with the largest fertility declines have pushed to provide information about contraception to both men and women and to provide women with the right to choose about their bodies; when they have this right, she is confident that they will take the proper precautions to have smaller families.

An assumption about the incompatible relationship between Islam and family planning underpins Zlotnik's comments and is woven throughout the arguments made in the best-selling book and popular article by Huntington and Goldstone, respectively: Islamic beliefs and practices and birth control—as a concept and as a method for population control—are contradictory to one another. Zlotnik conjectured that Islam is a barrier to the promotion and acceptance of reproductive healthcare and family planning. Muslim states need to overcome it in order to become modern, to provide resources for their citizens, and to ultimately compete economically on a global scale. However, the objective of this chapter is to challenge the assumption that being Muslim is not conducive to the acceptance of family planning and reproductive healthcare. In what follows, I give attention to both embodied and discursive practices of piety and reproduction with special consideration to how religious beliefs and economic reasoning for having or not having children converge in Moroccan women's everyday lives. On the one hand, I hope to convey how contraception is already pious in nature for many of the women who participated in my research and for medical providers. And on the other, I want to problematize this relationship by discussing the points of contradiction and contestation that they must navigate in accepting or providing reproductive health services.

## THE ABORTION DEBATE: CHOICES BETWEEN RELIGIOUS REPERCUSSIONS AND LIFE CIRCUMSTANCES

The abortion debate in Morocco serves as an example of how the intersection of religion, economics, and social discourses surrounding reproduction and the family is inscribed upon the bodies of Muslim women. A thirty-one-year-old woman, is quoted in a news magazine as saying, "I hope God can pardon me, but I couldn't bring this infant into the world, that would have had very serious consequences for my life." She had had three abortions at the time she was interviewed by the magazine. A second woman quoted in the article says, "I know that it's forbidden, but it is also forbidden to bring a child into this world who is not desired by his parents." She was only nineteen years old and had recently terminated an unplanned pregnancy. This article highlights the tension between religious questions surrounding abortion in Morocco and the everyday living conditions of the population. These quotes from the article illustrate their fear of possible repercussions they may face because they ended their pregnancies due to economic pressures and social expectations.

The abortion policy in Morocco punishes all medical professionals, other individuals who perform the procedure, and the women who receive it in times other than when it is necessary to save their lives (Population Division of the United Nations, n.d.). In cases of rape, incest, or sexual assault, abortion is not permissible.[3] In cases when the procedure is allowed, the doctor must first gain permission of the woman's spouse, father, or male guardian. If this is not possible, then the medical professional must seek the permission of the top state medical authority in the region (ibid.). The director of the RHO, Mr. Masjeel, stated in our interview, "Abortion constitutes a sanitary, social, and economic problem. It contributes to the high rate of maternal mortality in Morocco . . . it causes social problems in particular for young women between fifteen and thirty years of age." A small survey conducted in Morocco in 1984 found that four out of ten women interviewed had had an abortion. The researchers discovered that it was not uncommon for women to have up to three abortions in their lifetime (Hadley 1996). Islamic doctrines on abortion are not exactly clear, and, when taken in combination with social and economic forces of everyday life, they create a maze that women need to navigate in their reproductive decision making and practices.

The news article that quotes the two women also mentions that there has been a call for *ijtihad* over abortion, a process where legal decisions are made based upon interpretations of religious and legal sources (the Qur'an, Sunnah, and Hadith). *Ijtihad* is the interpretation of issues that are not directly addressed in the Qur'an or religious texts and is seen as a way to adapt Islam to a changing world.[4] Hajjer, the staff member at the RHO's main office, often pondered why poorer women in Morocco seemed to have more children than those who were wealthier. She explained that it is widely known and accepted in the country that Islam does not prohibit the use of contraception as long as it is not permanent. Hajjer said, "There are two things the Qur'an prohibits, abortion and sexual relations outside of marriage. Nothing else is forbidden in Islam." One spring morning in 2008, Hajjer and I shared a car ride with two other RHO staff members to the organization's youth festival in a nearby beach town. Hajjer mentioned the situation of a woman who had worked as a volunteer for the organization's outreach program in a smaller town in the Rabat region. This woman became pregnant and ended up terminating her pregnancy illegally. Hajjer made the comment to the other staff members that even in countries where abortion by choice is legal, the procedure is still not morally right.

Some feminist groups and women's rights activists are pushing for the legalization of abortion in Morocco under certain circumstances and within a specified time frame.[5] This time period is debated, but it would be between approximately forty and 120 days after conception, which is prior to the time when according to the Qur'an the fetus receives a soul (*ruh*) from God:[6] "We created man from an essence of clay, then We placed him as a drop of fluid in a safe place, then We made that drop into a clinging form, and We made that form into a lump of flesh, and We made that lump into bones, and We clothed those bones with flesh, and later We made him into other forms—glory be to God, the best of creators!" (23:12–14) Activists continue to lobby for abortion to be legal in cases of rape, incest, or when a family's economic circumstances would not be favorable for a child. In early 2012 the newly appointed Moroccan prime minister, Benkirane, from the PJD, stated he would support an initiative to allow abortions in cases of rape and incest. Mustapha Khalifi, the new communications minister, argued, "the government should push ahead with a proposal . . . to address the steep rise both in illegal abortions and in the number of unmarried mothers caught in the poverty trap" (Jay 2012).[7] Whereas moves have been made by activists and the government to make abortion more accessible and decriminalized in certain situations, fear of religious consequences and backlash continue to loom in the consciences of Moroccan citizens and policy makers.

## ISLAM AND ECONOMICS IN REPRODUCTIVE DECISION MAKING

The abortion debate is an example of when religious beliefs and practices play an equal or even greater role in people's reproductive decisions compared with social and economic circumstances. Faye Ginsburg, in her work on abortion in the United States, has suggested the procedure is a site of an emergent "life crisis" for women where they are often torn between "the conditions they faced—for example, become a mother—and the available cultural resources for structuring that change, cognitively and socially"

(1998, 13). Abortion serves as a node where various discourses, life forces, practices, emotions, and medical ethics meet. I found that popular Islamic understandings of reproduction and motherhood were mapped onto medical and social discourses by patients and medical staff at the health clinics where I conducted my research.

I want to argue against a utilitarian and totalizing view of religion that tends to be described by much of the literature on the relationship between health, religion, and economics (cf. Angrosino 2001; Garrity 2000; Henderson 2009). Instead, I adopt a line of thinking that is similar to Caroline Bledsoe and Fatoumatta Banja, who propose "reproductive capacity is measured . . . by individualized experiences of cumulative wearing traumatic events" (2002, 3). Following suit, rather than starting with religion as being opposed to economics, I find it more productive to conceptualize religious beliefs and practices as working in tandem with women's economic conditions to influence their reproductive decisions and behaviors. Whereas the debate surrounding religion and economics is not particularly new to scholarly endeavors on healthcare, it has become especially salient given the post-9/11 political focus on migration of poor Muslims to the West. Karl Marx addressed this debate. He writes:

> Man makes religion; religion does not make man. Religion is, in fact, the self-consciousness and the self-esteem of man who has either not yet gained himself or has lost himself again. But man is no abstract being squatting outside the world. Man is the world of man, the state, society. This state, this society, produce religion, which is an inverted world-consciousness, because they are an inverted world . . . [religion] is the opium of people. (1970, 131)

In this passage, Marx advocates that religion must be understood in relation to economics, politics, and the social worlds in which we live. Religion is dependent upon these forces as it "does not make man," but, rather, it is created through man's interactions and readings. Marx refers to religion as "the opium of people," which means that it has the ability to fill a void or to dull pain; however, it is not the cure for the actual ailment. Religion is described as allowing people to create a fantasy of the future, which then they are able to strive toward. However, they must try to change their circumstances instead of creating this future in their minds that is or is not attainable. Reading Marx in regards to the abortion debate in Morocco and to reproductive practices, we may conclude that when economic constraints come about, individuals will draw on religion to help them mediate these issues. In other words, religion is their "fallback" and not particularly a primary force that influences their decision making. Marx goes on to state that religion is "the heart of a heartless world, the soul of soulless conditions" and the "abolition of religion as the illusory happiness of a people is a demand for their true happiness" (1970, 131). Marx's theorization is valuable because it offers a way to conceptualize religion as plural given that "man makes religion" and it is dependent on systems of society; the form religion may take may look different depending on the context. But it does not provide a space for religion to be on an equivalent plane as economics and social circumstances. Religion is on the lower end of the hierarchy.

Recent studies of religion and individuals' use of healthcare services have built upon Marx's theorization of religious beliefs as being outside of the primary mode of decision making and practice (Jones 2004). For instance, Laurel Arthur Burton and Marcia Sue Dewolf Bosek argue, "Both spirituality and religion may be positively correlated with health outcomes . . . for religious people . . . the right decisions are clear because they, their beliefs and practices, have been *formed* in the structures of the particular religious community" (2000, 98; original italics). They suggest medical practitioners must be sensitive to religious objections to the treatment and be "respectful of religion as part of the context for care" (ibid.). However, Burton and Bosek consider religion to lie outside of the medical or scientific. Scholars of public health contend religion must be incorporated into medical treatment by staff, but it is circumscribed as something exceptional or separate from life circumstances (Body 2011; Daaleman and VandeCreek 2000). Loren Marks (2006) makes a recommendation that scholars ask four questions in research on religion and health decision making: What type of religion? What dimension of religion? What type of individual? And what type of health (social, psychological, biological)? I would like to suggest that we not only ask these questions, but we also analyze the process by which religion is brought together with medicine to form new discourses and practices within healthcare facilities and people's everyday lives.

Fertility rates have been shown to be in part contingent upon religious interpretations and social contexts (Sholkamy 1999). Comments made to me by a university student named Yassine reiterate this. I was a guest instructor in an undergraduate course on cross-cultural perspectives of gender at a university in Morocco, and our conversation that day turned to the relationship between religion and health practices, particularly those dealing with sexual and reproductive health. Yassine said that in the United States it is more about state law, actual guidelines will prohibit and allow certain practices, but in Morocco he believes it is more about people's mentalities, attitudes, and interpretations of Islam. A few students in the class who were from a large city in central Morocco, including Yassine, commented the local conservative ruling party there does not permit the sale of NorLevo (the "morning after" pill that helps prevent pregnancy after unprotected sexual intercourse) in pharmacies because of their strict religious beliefs. These college students do not see religion as being separate from the controversies surrounding NorLevo in their hometown, but rather religious beliefs are integral to the party's concern over sexual relations and the subsequent use of this pill.[8] Islamic doctrine is flexible when it comes to reproductive choices and can be manipulated with the intention to legitimize and reinforce contradictory positions concerning women and their reproductive bodies (Obermeyer 1995). In other words, Islam can be implored to either grant rights and liberties or take them away. As with the case of NorLevo, I turn now to how different understandings of what Islam says about reproduction and motherhood are intertwined with economic and social forces and medical discourses for the purpose of either promoting or prohibiting particular reproductive practices.

## IMAGES AND THE MESSAGES CONVEYED THROUGH THEM ABOUT ISLAM

As discussed in Chapter 2, when you walk into the clinics of the RHO, the first thing you notice is the multiple posters that line the walls of the waiting rooms. These posters illustrate powerful messages about sexual and reproductive health in addition to proper motherhood practices. One poster in particular caught my attention. It hung in both of the organization's health clinics in Tarma and Zitounia. The poster depicted a family in a living room area of a house. The mother is sitting on the couch with her husband and daughter nearby, and a little boy is playing on the floor at her feet. The daughter appears to be about six or seven years old, and the son is just a toddler. The woman wears a hijab and djellaba while she sews, and the husband is reading a book with the little girl. Over the mother's head there is a thought bubble that reads in Arabic, "The pill for protection from pregnancy, easy to use and effective." At the bottom of the poster against a dark blue background is a woman's hand holding a one-month supply of birth control pills. Next to this image there is a calendar with a date circled in red, reminding women that they must start a new cycle of pills each month in order for them to be effective. This was one of the biggest complaints that I heard from women in Morocco. They stated that they were not made aware they needed to take the pill month after month in order for it to work. When I visited a village in the Mid Atlas Mountains with members of a local aid organization, which had raised money to build an elementary school there, one woman explained that she had three children and decided to take the birth control pill so not to have another child. However, the medical provider did not tell her that she needed to come back each month for a new cycle of pills. She ended up pregnant with her fourth child, a boy, and was open about the fact that her pregnancy was unexpected, unplanned, and unwanted.

Two pictures that appeared in a textbook used in sexual and reproductive health classes at a local public school in Rabat were extremely provocative in their depictions of what the ideal Moroccan family should look like and the role that Islam plays in its creation. Given that my discussion is based on how these images frame Islam in relation to economics, I want to make a caveat here. In Morocco, citizens are automatically considered to be

Muslim because it is the national religion. It does not matter if an individual practices or not. Certain public sanctions are enforced for all Moroccan citizens based upon Islamic practices, such as no eating in the streets during the month of Ramadan, when Muslims are to fast from sunup to sundown with the exception of children, those who are ill, and women who are pregnant or menstruating.[9] Because of the prohibition of sex outside of marriage in Islam, women who become pregnant out of wedlock are often ostracized and shut out by their families. I point out these sanctions because I want to argue that Islamic beliefs and practices underlie these images and their interpretations even if they are not stated outright as such.

In the school textbooks, under the section about contraception there is a cartoonlike drawing of two families directly above a picture of different contraceptive methods. In the photo, two families are both standing in the rain. The one family has an umbrella, but there are too many children trying to stand underneath it at the same time. This leads to some of the children getting drenched by the water. The family has six children total, who appear to range in age from just a few months old to almost teenagers. The mother is wearing a long dress with a hijab, and the father dons a Moroccan djellaba and a turban. He also has a beard, which marks a true Muslim man for many countries in the Muslim world, including Morocco.[10]

The second family depicted in this pair consists of a man and woman with their two children. This is in stark contrast to the first image. The man is holding an umbrella while wearing a dapper suit. The mother is wearing a green pleated dress. In the first family, the parents wear clothing that has come to be associated with Islam in Morocco, but in this family, the mother has blond hair, which is not all that common in the country.[11] The mother in this family can be interpreted in a number of ways—a representation of colonial history of Morocco, a symbol of the continued presence of French and foreign nationals, or a depiction of the dream of many Moroccan men have of marrying a European or American woman to move out of the country. Regardless of how she is interpreted, the important thing here is to recognize the contrast between the two images and what messages they are giving off to young women in these sexual education classes about the relationship between Islam, economic circumstances, and reproduction.

## THE HIJAB, REPRODUCTION, AND CONTRADICTIONS

In the images from the RHO's clinics and the public school textbooks, the hijab is a main topic of interest because it points to the relationship between fertility and Islamic beliefs and practices. Whereas scholars have masterfully demonstrated that there are multiple meanings behind the hijab (Deeb 2006; Winter 2008), some of which link it to a notion of status or class rather than piety (Bullock 2002; Shirazi 2003), in Morocco, the hijab has come to be equated with a symbol of religious identity and emancipation.

Leila Ahmed (1992), in *Women and Gender and Islam*, traces the development of Islamic discourses surrounding women and their bodies both historically and geographically in order to show the socially constructed nature of gender within Muslim communities. She notes:

> What is or is not unique, specific, or intrinsic to Islam with respect to ideas about women and gender has already, then, become a complicated question. It is also clear that conceptions, assumptions, and social customs and institutions relating to women and to the social meaning of gender that derived from traditions in place in the Middle East at the time of Islamic conquests entered into and helped to shape the very foundations of Islamic concepts and social practice . . . All these facts emphasize the importance of considering Islamic formulations of gender in relation to the changing codes and practices in the broader Middle East. (1992, 5)

The inherent Islamic nature of the hijab is not static, but questionable, and it must be understood in the larger political, historical, and social context. In Morocco, the hijab has come to be seen as a marker of piety rather than as a representation of cultural constructions of gender or class. In the summer of 2008, young men and women who took part in a short class on sexual and reproductive health provided by the RHO in Agadir became engaged in a heated debate about Islam and violence against women. They all agreed that the violence women experience, such as harassment on the streets, is not due to Islam but is in part a result of people's religious interpretations and lack of education. However, one young man was adamant that women must dress modestly, including wearing the hijab, because it is in the Qur'an: "O Prophet, tell your wives and your daughters and the women of the believers to draw their cloaks close round them (when they go abroad). That will be better, so that they may be recognized and not annoyed. Allah is ever Forgiving, Merciful" (33:59).[12] A young woman responded by saying that she wears the hijab because she chooses to do so as a Muslim, not because she feels that she is compelled to do so. Within their exchange it was obvious there were differences between how this young woman and young man interpreted the meaning and purpose of the hijab, but both associated it with their Muslim identities.

Acclaimed Moroccan feminist scholar Fatima Sadiqi argues, "For many men, Islamist or not, the veil remains a sign of Islamic affiliation and traditional piety. For many women, however, the veil is a token of liberation—an indication that they have engaged with the Moroccan public in ways that reflect their own sense of religious practice" (2006). As I previously mentioned, in 2006, the Moroccan government removed photos of women and girls wearing the hijab from religious studies textbooks in public schools in addition to verses from the Qur'an that encourage women to cover their heads. (In addition, Royal Air Maroc, the state airline, has banned individuals from praying at their offices or headquarters because in the past, employees have supposedly abused the time they are allowed to pray.[13]) Although controversies surround the headscarf in many countries (Brems 2006; Olson 1985), until 2006 it was generally not a controversial issue in Morocco. The removal of pictures and verses was done because the government feared the hijab would be used as a symbol of Islamic extremism (Hamilton 2006). Verses from the Qur'an such as this one are no longer taught to young students:

> Enjoin believing women to turn their eyes away from temptation and to preserve their chastity; not to display their adornments (except such as are normally revealed); to draw their veils over their bosoms and not to display their finery except to their husbands, their fathers, their sons, their sisters' sons, their women-servants, and their slave-girls; male attendants lacking in natural vigor, and children who have no carnal knowledge of women. And let them not stamp their feet when walking so as to reveal their hidden trinkets. (4:31)

For the majority of women I engaged with during fieldwork, the hijab is seen as a marker of piety. Hajjer asked me one day about a family we were both mutual acquaintances of. She asked me about the three daughters of the household and whether or not they left the home frequently besides going to school. I said that the girls tended to do chores around the home or watch television whereas the two sons went out with their friends to play soccer or just hang out. Hajjer said, "Her husband is very Muslim. He and his wife have some problems. Is she Muslim? Does she wear the [hijab]?[14] I think she does." She made a connection between the seclusion of the daughters to their father's Islamic beliefs and made the assumption that if she wears the hijab, then she is a practicing Muslim. Hajjer's concern and comments demonstrate the hijab is a sign of piety in Morocco. This allows for a connection to be made between Islamic understandings and the concepts of fertility and motherhood in my analysis of images given that the women in the photos tend to be wearing hijabs.

A second vignette that illustrates this relationship comes from my interview with Dr. Binjal. While discussing the RHO's health clinics, he asked me if I noticed the counselors or female physicians wearing the hijab while providing medical services. When I responded that I had, he replied with the following:

> This what [the founders] didn't want. When [the clinic staff] wear the veil, they do not just cover their heads, the only thing they do is cover their brains. I do not believe that religion should be a question. I think that we need to take it out of the picture altogether. Religion should not be mixed with politics or the government. The women who wear the veil don't help the patients at the clinic.

What Dr. Binjal meant in his comments was that piousness has caused the medical staff to not be objective when providing health services to patients. He assumes that their religious beliefs and practices cloud their medical judgments and opinions. The hijab, which he saw as being a marker of a Muslim woman, was equated with stricter ideas about gender, the family, and women's bodies. Islam and medical care are not to be mixed because such a dangerous mixture would not facilitate improving care or advancing women's rights over their reproductive bodies. However, the image from the poster in the health clinics contradicts Dr. Binjal's assumptions about the incompatibility of religion and healthcare. The family does not appear to be poor nor does the mother have a sad look on her face as in the images from the school textbooks. Her children are not wearing tattered clothing, and they are not malnourished, also complicating the link between poverty and Muslim identity seen in popular culture and the schoolbooks in Morocco. Rather, the woman and her family appear to be content in their living room sewing, playing, or reading. I offer an interpretation of this picture that draws on Sadiqi's argument. The mother of this particular family, with her dress demonstrating piety, is engaged with some of the key themes of development and Islam in Morocco, such as self-regulation and providing a quality life for the family. She controls her fertility through the regular use of contraception. For her, as for many women who came into the clinics over the course of my fieldwork, contraception is already a pious practice because it represents ethical ideals of Islam that surround the body, family, motherhood, and reproduction.

The family is overwhelmed by children in the second set of images I described taken from the school textbooks (with the woman wearing a hijab and the man wearing a turban). This picture represents the problematic link between piety and poverty. The woman is not portrayed as using a method of contraception given the manner in which she and her husband are shown: weary, frustrated, tired, and hopeless. The second family (with the woman wearing a dress and the husband in a suit) is happy with just two children and is able to take care of them. It is assumed that they controlled their reproductive bodies and fertility through the use of contraception. However, if the hijab is a marker of female Muslim identity in Morocco, then it may also be assumed that this woman is not a practicing Muslim. This portrays disjuncture between being a Muslim and making responsible reproductive decisions—the two seem to be incompatible in this particular image.

## ISLAM AND FAMILY PLANNING: CONTRACEPTION AS A PIOUS PRACTICE

The Qur'an does not explicitly or implicitly discuss contraception, leaving the matter up for interpretation (Keefe 2006). The relationship between

Islam and family planning is not clear-cut, which points to the question of what extent Islam is monolithic and homogenous given that Muslims live in various social, political, and cultural contexts (Bowen 2004). Because Islam has no central authority over all Muslims, like the Vatican has over Catholics around the world, multiple interpretations and local expectations exist for Islamic beliefs and practices, including the use of contraception.

In Islam, marriage and having children is not a requirement, but it is of particular importance for "stabilizing community mores, organizing family structure, and averting the social chaos that could result from unregulated sexual contact" (Bowen 2004, 121). An Imam reiterated this to me when I interviewed him at a mosque in the Mid Atlas Mountains. He stated that the family was the foundation of a Muslim society, and he also explained that a man could marry a woman who was infertile or a couple could choose not to have children because "the goal of marriage is love and mercy" not procreation.[15] In addition, both the husband and wife have a say in determining the number of children and the spacing of births in order to promote the health of the mother and the economic and social well-being of the family (Bowen 2004). Islam is not separate from everyday life for a believer, and proper behaviors in all domains of a person's life, including reproductive practices, can be realized by referencing religious texts and debates.

Often Islam is seen as prohibiting the use of modern contraceptives (Bop 2005; Degni et al. 2008) precisely because the Qur'an does not address family planning (Esposito 2002). Carla Makhlouf Obermeyer (1995) argues that Islamic doctrine is often "invoked" with the intention to legitimize and reinforce contradictory positions in the MENA concerning women and their reproductive bodies. However, jurists of the Maliki School of Islam,[16] the jurisprudence the majority of Moroccans follow, even confirm that *al-'azl* (withdrawal) is allowed in marriage with the consent of the wife and some even go as far to argue that she must be compensated if she agrees to practice coitus interruptus (Omran 1992). This is the only method of contraception that is mentioned in religious texts. The hadith recounted by Jabir Ibn Abdullah states, "[The companions of the Prophet] used *'azl* during the time of the Prophet while the Qur'an was being revealed" (quoted in Bowen 2004, 128) Another similar version of this says, "We used to practice *'azl* during the time of the Prophet. The Prophet came to know about it, but did not forbid us" (ibid.). Whereas debate surrounds the use of modern methods of contraception in the Muslim world, the vast majority of jurists have agreed that methods such as the birth control pill or IUD are permissible as long as they do not destroy a person's ability to have children. Modern methods are actually looked upon more favorably in some cases because they do not disrupt normal sexual relations inside of marriage (Omran 1992).

Across the Muslim world and even inside communities there are several interpretations of what Islam says about reproduction and fertility (Inhorn

2005; Johnson-Hanks 2006a). Medical anthropologists have made note of this in their work on individuals' experiences of reproduction and fertility in Muslim communities. Sargent discusses the moral conflicts that Muslim Malian migrants who have settled in France face when they come in contact with the French healthcare system. Sargent argues, "Malian women and men frame reproductive decisions and discourses in diverse interpretations of Islam as they seek to manage the contradictions of everyday life in France and assert individual agency" (2006, 32). Also, Susi Krehbiel Keefe learned in her work among African Muslim women in Tanzania that "religious (Islamic) values and reproductive reasoning are fashioned pragmatically in this context. Individuals in Ugweno construct reproductive lives that challenge overly deterministic understandings of the relationship between religion and contraceptive practices" (2006, 419). Even though sterilization is generally seen as going against Islam's position that it is not permissible to stop childbearing permanently, women in Keefe's research manipulated Islamic understandings in order to justify their decisions to undergo the procedure. Whereas the Qur'an does not forbid sterilization outright, the permanent nature of the procedure has led many Muslim jurists to not permit it as a method of family planning (Stephenson 2006).

In a similar vein, in my own research, I discovered that female patients who visited the health clinics often used their Islamic beliefs to rationalize their use of contraception in order to limit the number of births or to space their children appropriately. Women often drew on religious and medical discourses in addition to their everyday life circumstances to account for their decisions to accept particular reproductive practices. More specifically, the majority of the patients who visited the clinics were of working-class status and did not have the financial or physical resources to provide for a number of children. Whereas women may have felt pressure coming from their familial and social networks to have a larger number of children, many of them justified not doing so through couching their decisions to accept contraception within their own Islamic understandings of reproduction.

## "LIFE IS HARD": RATIONALIZING THE USE OF CONTRACEPTION USING ISLAMIC BELIEFS

Nawal came to the RHO's clinic for an ultrasound wearing a gray abaya[17] and matching niqab.[18] She was five months pregnant with her second child, a boy. Even though her abaya was to protect her body from the male gaze, you could easily spot her growing "baby bump" protruding through the material. Nawal and her husband already had a little girl, who was five years old. I was able to follow Nawal throughout the majority of her second pregnancy. She returned to the clinic every month for a checkup and ultrasound. This was more than the providers recommended, but Nawal was being extra careful. She was twenty-six years old and had been married for six years. Her husband worked odd jobs in the construction business in the local area, and she remained at home to raise their daughter, who was at school the majority of days when she came to the clinic, although I was able to meet the young girl a few times over the course of my fieldwork. Whereas Nawal longed to return to her hometown outside of Fes, about a three-hour train ride from Rabat, her marriage had been arranged to her distant cousin and they settled near his family to raise their children. She had finally come to the realization that she would not be able to return to her hometown to live near her natal family, but she continued to hope for this prospect.

Nawal was excited about having her second child and was especially happy it was a boy. She was proud of the fact that she had waited to have a second child and was also relieved given how much energy she expends taking care of her daughter and husband. Nawal spaced her children by using the birth control pill. I asked why she thought it was best to wait. She responded that giving birth is difficult and raising a child can make a woman very tired. Even though she does not work outside of the home, she was always busy around the house cooking, cleaning, doing laundry, and running after her daughter. In addition to this, although her husband had a job in the local area, his career was not certain. There was little security in the construction business. She said, "*al-hayat ṣ'ba* " or "life is hard" over and over again during our many conversations, but despite the everyday difficulties to make ends meet, Nawal went on to explain to me that for all Muslims (regardless if one is a man or woman), children are a very important part of life. She stated one afternoon as we sat outside waiting for the doctor to arrive at the RHO's clinic:

> I love my daughter. I love my family. I love being a mother. For us, for Muslims, children are the heart of life. Children are very important for everyone. I like it when my daughter comes home from school. She says, "Mama, I learned this today in school," and she will show me her papers. I am so happy because I did not go to school like she does. I am very happy because she is happy.

As we sat together, I asked her to clarify why children are so important for Muslims. Nawal responded that God wants Muslims (both men and women) to have children, but he does not want them to have more children than they can actually provide for. It struck me that she said *al-mslmin* (the plural of Muslim in *darija*) meaning all Muslims as opposed to stating that children are important for just female believers or just male believers. Nawal's comments reminded me of a verse from the Qur'an that several women made reference to, including Fatima. It states, "God provides everyone out of His abundance, for God is resourceful, wise" (4:130). For them, this verse meant that God is astute and aware of people's everyday circumstances. He knows what is happening in their lives and will care for them accordingly. Although God understands what believers can and cannot handle financially, physically, and emotionally, Nawal implied that they must still act responsibly and make decisions that will better themselves and their families in order to live a proper Muslim life.

A friend of mine named Azhar, who is originally from Fes and works at a university, pointed out a second verse from the Qur'an that references childbearing. It reads:

> Say, Come let me tell you what your Lord has really prohibited for you: You shall not set up idols besides Him. You shall honor your parents. *You shall not kill your children from fear of poverty—we provide for you and for them.* You shall not commit gross sins, obvious or hidden. You shall not kill—*GOD has made life sacred*—except in the course of justice. These are His commandments to you that you may understand. (6:151; italics added)

This verse stipulates that individuals are not to kill their children "from fear of poverty." Likewise, Nawal suggested that men and women need to control their fertility in order to make the most out of their resources. In our conversation Nawal was adamant that children must have food, clothing, and love from their parents until they reach an age when they can provide for themselves. (Love continues beyond this point in time.) For her, not being able to give these things to your children or not having the means to offer them a good life would reflect poorly on the parents as Muslims. What Nawal did was create a link between providing for children and the degree to which a person is a proper Muslim. Whereas economic circumstances and the lack of job security for her husband played a role in her choice to delay her second pregnancy, Nawal couched these reasons in her own interpretations of Islamic teachings about fertility and motherhood.

## ISSUES IN ACCESSING CARE: FINANCE AND GENDER HIERARCHIES

Physicians who worked at the clinics were not immune to the confluence of religious and medical discourses with their patients' economic circumstances, such as those of Nawal. We must realize that all humans, whether they are patients or providers, "are products of their environment as well as its creators; therefore any consideration of the individual independent of his relationships and communities is self-defeating" (Gaylin 1996, 44). Several of the physicians at the RHO's clinics who allowed me to observe their work discussed how these multiple factors regularly influenced their medical practices. Their work is not divorced from the messy and intricate mix of religious beliefs, financial needs, and public health discourses in Morocco, but rather they too had to delicately negotiate it just like their patients.

Dr. Looz works full-time at a local hospital as an OB/GYN and spends one afternoon a week at the RHO's health clinic in Tarma and another afternoon at a second RHO clinic in Rabat. We sat one afternoon at the makeshift desk in the exam room talking before she started seeing the twenty-something patients that came to the clinic that day for her services. She was dressed in a white lab coat, a button-down shirt, and trousers. Her brown wavy hair was loose and looked a bit unkempt, a telltale sign of her busy afternoon schedule traveling from one facility to the next for work. I asked Dr. Looz to talk about the problems she faces in her practice on a regular basis. She could not come up with any issues related to her work off the top of her head, but after a minute or two of pondering she said that one major problem is that of *l'argent* or money. Dr. Looz stressed that this was of particular importance for the women in the local area of Tarma, who tended to be of lower socioeconomic statuses. Women and men were unable to afford the health services they needed, which is why it was so important for the RHO to subsidize its services for patients. Dr. Looz explained that financial problems are compounded by the fact that some women are unable to see the doctor or come to the clinic because of gender hierarchies in the household. She impersonated a man who she described as being the typical Moroccan husband: "Ninety percent of men in Morocco do not help with children. Women do it all. They take care of children, clean the house, and cook. A man will sit in his chair and say to his wife, 'Bring me a glass of water!' He won't get it himself. He wants her to do it. Women have no time." For her, seeing a doctor in the clinic may actually disrupt the gender roles and ideals within the household that have come to be seen as normalized and even routine in some families.

The Moroccan government, along with development organizations and even the media, encourages women to use contraception in order to regulate their pregnancies and to seek out maternal healthcare when they are pregnant. However, as Dr. Looz observes, this may not be possible for all Moroccan women, which may cause them not to live up to the government's expectations of modern citizens. During our conversation, Dr. Looz also mentioned that the ways some individuals interpret Islamic tenets in terms of masculine and feminine roles in the family have placed restrictions on women's movements and choices. These particular interpretations do not permit women to enter the public spaces of the medical facility for proper care, and, therefore, economics is not the only reason women may not be able to seek medical services. Economic conditions are confounded with religious interpretations of gender. The paradox that Amina Wadud (1999) describes in her examination for the creation story in the Qur'an resonates with the hindrances experienced by Dr. Looz in her work. Wadud argues that despite differences in the treatment of men and women in the creation of humankind, there are not any "essential differences in the value attributed to women and men" (1999, 15). In this framework then, health and well-being are rights of both sexes regardless of religious sanctions placed on certain behaviors of men and women.

## CONCLUSION: ISLAM, INTERPRETATIONS, AND PROVIDING HEALTHCARE

Similar to Dr. Looz, Dr. Mamouri also stated that he faced a problem in his work that concerned gender hierarchies in the home. When I interviewed him in his cramped hospital office while sipping on orange tea with him, he said:

> I do not have many problems [in my work]. The only problem I have is the extremists, the Islamists. You know the men with beards and women who wear the veil. Sometimes the men don't allow their wives to see me because I'm a man. They see a man. They don't see a doctor. The women don't care. They don't have problems, but men cannot separate the man and the doctor. This is bad for the woman's health. But that is the only barrier in my work.

It is not Islam that hinders Dr. Mamouri's practice as a doctor; rather, it is the Islamists in Morocco, according to him. Religion is not the problem. He attributes the contradictions that prevent women from using contraception or receiving care in a medical facility to those who may be termed more "conservative" Muslims because they are unable to separate the doctor from the man. If "conservative" men would allow their wives, sisters, or daughters to see him for care, it would violate their religious understandings about opposite sex interactions.

The issues that Dr. Looz and Dr. Mamouri face in their work point to the fact that reproductive healthcare, popular Islamic understandings, and discourses of development cannot be separated from people's everyday economic circumstances, women's identity formation, and constructions of gender within the family. I argue that something new is being produced where such domains cannot be distinguished from one another. New "conjugations" (Bracke 2008; Deeb 2009) are created that bring these discourses, practices, and life circumstances together. Islam is just one piece of the complicated development puzzle, and particular religious interpretations actually aid to the production of responsible and modern Moroccan citizens who regulate their fertility, such as in the case of Nawal. What I have hoped to show in this chapter is that Islam is not incompatible with family planning as a religion, but different interpretations are possible given that it is not monolithic or homogenous. Whereas some of these interpretations may cause problems for physicians in their work, as discussed by Dr. Looz and Dr. Mamouri, others, such as the Islam that is depicted in the poster at the RHO clinic, encourage the use of medical practices to control fertility and enhance personal well-being. Instead of fearing Muslim fertility and thinking of it as a potential "population bomb" (Ehrlich 1968; Goldstone 2010), we need to better understand the nuances of Islamic beliefs and practices of reproduction in addition to Muslims' actual experiences. The next chapter continues this discussion through an examination of rapid pregnancy tests that were given in the RHO clinics and seeks to demonstrate that female patients oftentimes rationalized the test results through a discussion of how God understands what they can and cannot handle in their lives. Similar to this chapter, Chapter 5 also shows how women placed the religious on an equal plane as economics, medical discourses, scientific facts, and their everyday circumstances.

# 5 "I Can't, God Knows It"
## Pregnancy Tests and Islamic Rationality

> There were several women at the clinic for a pregnancy test. The intern took care of them. She called them into the counseling room but then Kaoutar told them to wait outside. It was a bit confusing at the moment. The one woman was born in 1976, which makes her 33 years old. Her test was negative. She was happy! Another woman in a light blue veil, which covered her completely, also had a negative result. She left the room immediately after this. I didn't quite make out what the result of the 26-year-old woman's test was, but the 23-year-old woman who wore a yellow djellaba also had a negative pregnancy test. No women were pregnant today! I asked the intern if this was correct and she said it was. So obviously the woman whose test I didn't see wasn't pregnant as well. (Excerpt from field notes February 19, 2009)

At the RHO's clinics, women lined up each morning for rapid pregnancy tests, and their reactions to the test results illustrated the intimate relationship between Islam, economics, and responsibility. One of the first questions that the directors Kaoutar and Fatima posed to women when they wanted to have a pregnancy test was how long they had been married. This question echoes the critique made by religious scholars and Muslims in Morocco about the main goal of marriage being procreation, when in fact this is not so any longer. A 1995 publication by the RHO originally stated that the objective of marriage for Muslims was to have children, but the organization later revised this statement in its more recent Plan of Action. After the clinical staff went through the process of the pregnancy test, they wrote *positif* or *negatif* on a slip of paper and handed it to the women. On numerous occasions, women would repeat "Alhamdulillah," meaning, "Thanks be to God" over and over again when they saw negative results.[1] The vast majority of women who were told they were not pregnant would quickly leave the counseling room with smiles on their faces. They were happy and praising God that they were not expecting.

Their reactions contradict much of what has been written about pregnancy and children in Morocco and highlight the changing ideas of motherhood in recent decades. Scholars have suggested children hold an incredibly valuable place in women's imaginaries and are important for how women are defined within Moroccan society (Bowen 1993; Dwyer 1978). Whereas scholarship does not argue that having as many children as possible is the ideal, it has reiterated the significance of large families in the past as a way for women to build their social status. In her study or rural Moroccan women, Bourqia (1995) notes that working-class and poorer women in Morocco are hesitant to accept family planning because they depend on their children to provide for them in the future. In addition, giving birth helps define women's existence in the family and community and helps to give them a place in society and social status. This line of thinking held true in several conversations I had with older Moroccan women. They expressed the need for their children to help support them in whatever way possible, even though it may not be much. For many of these women, the willingness to help their parents or their recognition of being indebted was a crucial attribute that children are to possess. For example, I met Hadal when I visited the women's weaving co-op in which she participated. There was no middleman for the co-op, so Hadal was able to keep 100 percent of the profits from the sales of her rugs instead of giving money to a person between her and the buyer. After purchasing one of her rugs, I asked Hadal what she does with the money. Hadal is diabetic and purchases medication with the money. Some of the funds will go towards household goods and to buy more yarn to weave rugs and blankets. She will give the rest of the money to her four sons who live in the same village. She stated that she gives them money because prior to her participation in the weaving co-op and earning income, her sons helped take care of her and her husband by providing financially for them. In a way, this is her repayment to her children for helping her economically, before she was able to make some money of her own through selling rugs. She said to me about her sons, "They

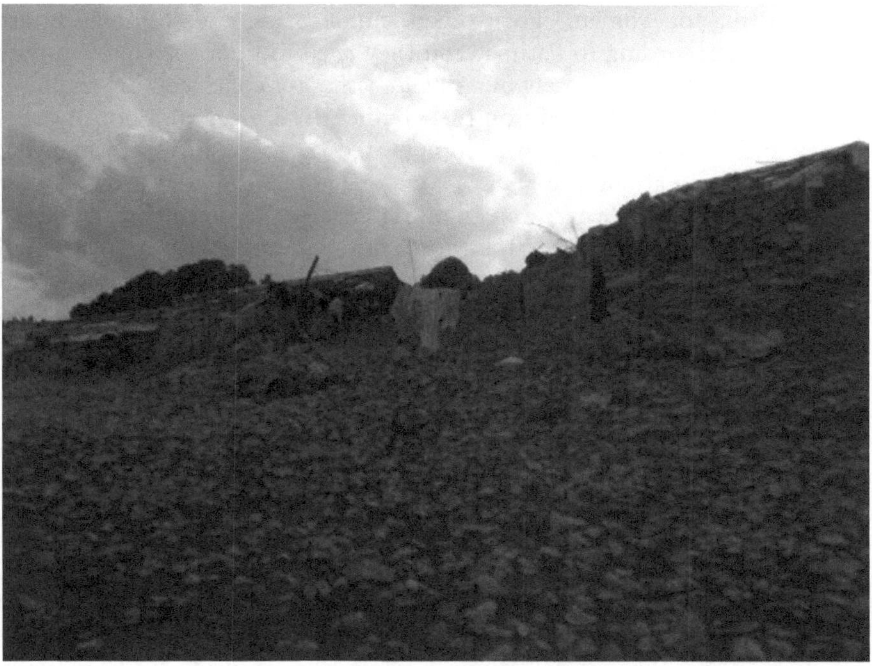

*Figure 5.1* The village of a weaving cooperative. (Photo by the author).

are good boys." However, in contrast, many women at the RHO clinics were overjoyed to learn they were not expecting. This does not mean they are not good mothers as compared to some of the other women I interacted with, who stated outright that children were a very important part of their lives. Rather, it demonstrates evolving notions of motherhood that have come with the implementation of neoliberal development programs, notably the INDH, and emphasizes the convergence of medical and religious discourses concerning childbearing and childrearing occurring in women's daily lives.

Women's responses to their pregnancy tests often combined their religious beliefs with their economic constraints. After negative tests, several women expressed concern that they physically not could care for a child (whether their first or an addition) because their bodies could not handle it. Fatima echoed this sentiment several times while counseling patients on the importance of using contraception. One afternoon a gentleman came to the RHO clinic in Tarma dressed in a suit and tie. He was middle-aged and had slightly graying hair. I found out later that he worked for the local government, which sometimes did checks on the clinic unexpectedly. He asked Fatima about the services the clinic offered to women. She discussed all of the different methods of contraception and even took the poster off the wall of the counseling room that had the various methods taped to it (birth control pills, male condoms, IUDs, etc.). While discussing the methods with the gentleman, he asked her why women should use contraception. Fatima responded that "giving birth makes a woman tired" and "raising children is very tiring for women." For women, childbearing and childrearing are exhausting, according to Fatima, and they need to limit their pregnancies and space them appropriately by using a method of contraception so not to put too much physical strain on their bodies. The physical labor of pregnancy and raising children was complicated by the reality that many of the women who attend the RHO's clinic may not be able to provide their children with adequate care and all of life's necessities given their working-class backgrounds. Several of the Moroccan women I observed, who I will discuss in this chapter, even stated that God understood this and would only give them what they could handle. This is why their pregnancy tests were negative, not because conception did not take place.

This chapter discusses how women negotiated believing in the scientific aspects of pregnancy, such as how the rapid pregnancy test works, with their beliefs in God's will and their understandings of Islam. As I sat in the counseling room with Fatima and Kaoutar, I noticed that women often called upon God after they received their desired or undesired results, which shows how the boundaries between medical and religious discourses surrounding the reproductive body are obliterated in the clinical space. The biological and the scientific do not exist separately from their religious beliefs and spirituality. The female participants in my research turned the assumption that the medical trumps God or religion inside out by actually merging the two together. The pregnancy test, a medical practice that is supposed to contribute to the creation of modern reproductive subjects and citizens, has taken on a very new meaning for these women. The state and the medical community in Morocco have encouraged women to begin to seek maternal healthcare as soon as possible after their positive pregnancy test. Whereas the test serves the same function across the board (i.e., to determine pregnancy at five or six weeks after conception), for the women I observed, it also becomes a way for them to make "belief statements" (Kirsch 2004). Lisa Ann Richey argues that in large-scale surveys, the "desire for children is measured as a dichotomous variable (i.e., the pregnancy was wanted or unwanted)" (2008, 176), but the use of ethnographic methods that elicit women's stories can help us understand that pregnancies are not always "wanted" or "unwanted." There is a great deal of gray area in between these two desires. My observations of women's reactions to the results of their pregnancy tests combined with my informal interviews suggest that the desire to become pregnant or not to become pregnant is complicated. In women's reactions, I could see that their understandings of what Islam says about fertility and motherhood converged with medical discourses of the body, scientific facts, and their everyday social and economic circumstances.

## TAKING A PREGNANCY TEST

On a typical weekday, I would arrive at the RHO's clinics in Tarma or Zitounia around 8:00 a.m. Fatima or Kaoutar would usually be checking women in at the time. The staff tended to arrive a little before 8:00 a.m. The clinics were much busier in the spring and fall than the summer and winter. This is because the vast majority of women either walked or took public transportation to get there. In the summer, the Rabat region tends to get very warm and humid, and in the winter, it can experience quite cold temperatures and sometimes snow. These conditions made it difficult for the patients to make it to the clinics during certain times of the year without a car. When I arrived, I would usually find about ten women in the waiting rooms. They had either been checked in already or were waiting to be seen by Fatima or Kaoutar. The RHO does not particularly advertise publicly; it relies on word of mouth to promote the services that it offers.[2] This word travels fast and quite far. Some women would travel a few hours just to come to the clinic for a rapid pregnancy test.

All of the RHO's clinics offer rapid pregnancy tests for thirty dirhams, which is roughly US$3.55. The pregnancy test is a plastic stick upon which the counselor would place a small amount of urine in a tiny hole.[3] Within a few minutes, lines would appear in the window, which is no more than one centimeter long. Each test is individually wrapped. They are manufactured in Germany and actually do not include instructions in French or Arabic, but rather only in German and English. I discovered this one morning when a substitute counselor was in for Fatima. The woman had not worked that often at the RHO clinic and was unfamiliar with the test procedure. When she asked me how it worked, I tried to show her the directions on the package, only to find that they were not in a language that she could read. I ended up translating the instructions to her so that she did it correctly to get an accurate result. The headquarters of the RHO has an employee, a young man in his mid to late thirties named Morad, who is strictly in charge of making sure each clinic has enough supplies. The directors take inventory of the clinic's supplies at the end of each month and submit a formal request for more supplies as needed. While I was conducting fieldwork, helping with inventory became a part of my routine and I often spent afternoons counting packages of birth control pills or the number of male condoms and pregnancy tests in an exam room at the RHO clinic in Tarma or Zitounia.

Fatima and Kaoutar would only administer the tests in the morning, and so women who wanted to know whether or not they were pregnant would line up outside of the clinic's doors before they even arrived. This is due to the fact that hormone levels in urine from the morning are higher and the test will be more accurate in the early part of the day rather than the later afternoon. Most pregnancy test makers recommend that first morning urine be used because it typically contains higher concentrations of hCG, the pregnancy hormone.[4] The higher levels will help prevent false negative results. If women came too late in the day, then they would often be turned away and told to come again the following morning. However, women did not give a urine sample at the clinic. Instead, they were required to bring their own samples, and usually they did so in a glass jar, which they wrapped in a plastic bag. This meant that women did not have to bring their own samples, but they could bring that from relatives or friends to be tested. I observed this quite often. One morning an older woman came in with another woman who appeared to be in her early to midthirties to the clinic in Zitounia. I sat with them in the counseling room as Kaoutar carefully took a drop of urine from the jar and placed it on the stick. As she filled out the paperwork and charted the services, the women revealed that it was not from one of them. They had brought a sample from their son/brother's wife. They left the room while Kaoutar checked in other patients. She then called them back to tell them the test was negative. They looked at each other, disappointed, but then said, "We'll be back in a few months to try again" before leaving the clinic. A mother-in-law or sister-in-law frequently brought in samples from her son's or brother's wife, which emphasizes the central role that a husband's family members continue to play in the couple's reproductive decision making and practices.

When women requested a pregnancy test, they would need to answer a set of questions. Besides the basic information, such as name, age, and place of residence, Fatima and Kaoutar would also inquire as to their marital status, number of children, and number of months or years between then and their most recent birth. If a woman thought she was pregnant for the very first time, they would ask how long it had been since she was married. I noticed Fatima in particular was a bit more critical of the women's answers to this question. On the one hand, if a woman answered that she had been married a year or more, Fatima would state that it was the right time to begin having children. If she had been married for longer than that, Fatima would inquire how long they had been trying (either intentionally or unintentionally, i.e., not doing anything to prevent a pregnancy but not actively trying either) to have children and why they had waited so long since their wedding. On the other hand, if a woman was younger and just married a few months, Fatima would encourage her to wait a little longer before beginning to have children. For her, there was a set time period when it was best to begin growing their families depending upon the woman's age at the time she came to the clinic and her age when she was married.

Melvin Konner (1993) reminds us that it is important to understand how physicians and medical staff are trained and socialized and how this impacts the delivery of care. A 1995 report produced by domestic and international development agencies stated that "procreation is a goal of marriage" and that "marriage and procreation are anchored tightly in the dominant mentality in Morocco" due to the prescriptions put forth by the *Moudawana.* Fatima's questions echo this sentiment; however, the publication also states that women must be protected by their husbands and provided security when they have children because being a woman and mother is symbolic for them in society. In her questioning prior to administering a pregnancy test, Fatima was also careful to inquire what the patient wanted at the time for herself and her family. She took into account the patient's reproductive desires to make the best recommendations for care.

After Fatima and Kaoutar took a drop of urine and placed it on the testing stick, the women would exit the counseling room and wait for their results. Usually within five or ten minutes, they would call the women back into the room to tell them if they were *ḥamla* or *ma ḥamla-sh*, pregnant or not pregnant. They would record the results, either *positif* or *négatif* on slip of paper with the patient's name, the date, and the RHO's official stamp and then hand it to her. They would also record the result in their record book. Theoretically, this is to be done in private so that no one can know a particular patient's results except the staff member and the patient, but this was not always the case. I observed on numerous occasions that the staff will do mass pregnancy tests. Women come in one by one and the tests are kept separate, but there may be five of six of them lying on Fatima's or Kaoutar's desk waiting to be read. (If Fatima and Kaoutar had multiple tests to read, they would put the slip of paper with each woman's name on it under the appropriate test. They would then record the results on this paper and return it to the patient.) The counselors often called women in to receive their results as other patients were packing up their things to leave the room and thus they were able to also hear whether or not the patient was indeed pregnant.

Conflicts often occurred between patients and staff when women wanted ultrasounds immediately instead of having a pregnancy test. This is just one way that the medical professionals continued to "negotiate control" over female patients' bodies with the intention of producing healthy future Moroccan citizens. I argue that it works to show how women's bodies are the vehicles through which the nation is produced. Ultrasounds are provided at the RHO's clinics in addition to maternity hospitals and private clinics in Morocco. Eugenia Georges (1996) observed that doctors in Greece will often offer multiple, sometimes unnecessary, ultrasounds to attract patients to the hospital so that they can keep them under the medical gaze. But in Morocco, medical providers at the RHO clinics silenced women's desires for ultrasounds instead of pregnancy tests because it violates the protocol and is viewed as "pathological" within this context. When staff obliged female patients who wanted ultrasounds right away instead of a pregnancy test, they were often lectured or reprimanded for their decisions.

I spoke with Dr. Mamouri about this issue. He stated that sometimes women are unsure as to when they should utilize the services at the clinics or hospitals. I found certain women did not trust the accuracy of the rapid tests, which was understandable given they were just small plastic strips. Other patients did not know that they should have brought urine samples with them. If they had traveled a long way to the clinic, they would not want to return another day, but they had no choice but to do so. Some women would request to have an ultrasound performed immediately to find out if they were pregnant. Fatima and Kaoutar would tell them that it was a waste of their time and money because an ultrasound costs three times as much as a pregnancy test at one hundred dirhams. A test could do the same quickly and accurately, but if the patients insisted, then they would arrange for the procedure right away.

At the RHO clinic, Dr. Mamouri came into the counseling room after he had seen a patient who requested an ultrasound instead of a pregnancy test. She was not pregnant. He sat on Fatima's desk; I was in the chair just a few feet away. He told her that he did not understand why women wanted an ultrasound because if they were not pregnant, all he could do was sign the chart and tell them to come back in the future if there was an issue. Of course if he had found something on the ultrasound, he would treat it immediately or refer the patient to the local hospital. But in this woman's case, he just told her to return if she experienced any problems, and she was very upset by this. Dr. Mamouri recounted this incident and just shook his head as Fatima explained that she tried to make this point to the woman when she checked her in that morning. She stated, "I told her you take the pregnancy test first. It's good. The test will say positive or negative. She didn't listen. She wanted an ultrasound. I said okay and took her money." After Fatima finished talking, Dr. Mamouri looked at me and said, "Crazy citizens!" He then proceeded to jump off the desk and storm out of the room. He returned to the exam room to continue seeing patients. Although

Dr. Mamouri was upset, he was not particularly angry with the woman, but rather with the broader system of healthcare in Morocco. It does not provide women with the information they need to make informed decisions about their bodies and reproductive lives. In our interview at his office, he said the Ministry of Health does not always offer counseling or informational sessions: "Women come here with information that is wrong. The information is stupid. They think the pill does X when it doesn't. They don't know, but it's not their fault. The Ministry doesn't help them." His comments point to the difficulty some women face in making choices about reproduction and their general health given the lack of resources they have to draw upon and their subsequent lack of health knowledge.

In the remaining sections of this chapter, I will focus specifically on women's reactions to their pregnancy tests and try to understand how their religious beliefs culminate around this relatively recent medical intervention. What I hope to show is how women's understandings of what Islam says about fertility and reproduction are malleable and transform as they come into contact with medical discourses and practices, and, at the same time, I hope to demonstrate that the medical and scientific facts, which tend to be considered objective and nonnegotiable, also are morphed as they interact with women's religious beliefs.

## BELIEVING AND ACTING: WOMEN'S REACTIONS TO THEIR PREGNANCY TESTS

After women receive a negative pregnancy test result, they are to be counseled by either Fatima or Kaoutar. This session is to include a discussion of contraception and the various methods that the clinics offer. During our interview one afternoon in the spring of 2008, I asked Fatima to explain to me what happens after a negative result and the patient does not want to become pregnant. What will she talk to her about? I wanted to know the specific conversation she would have with the woman in this particular situation. She explained to me:

> If a woman comes in for a pregnancy test and she is not pregnant then I ask her if she is using contraception. If she is, then I talk to her about the method and possibly changing methods because maybe it is not working. If she is not using a contraceptive method, then I insist [*insister*] that she uses a method. She must use one. She can choose the method she wants.

Women have a choice as to the specific contraceptive method they would like to use if they do not want to become pregnant at that time. It is assumed that in these cases, women are not using contraception if they believe that they may be expecting. Kaoutar's response was similar to that of Fatima's except she was not as forceful in her insistence that women use contraception. She would instead make a strong recommendation that women use a method of contraception or change the method. Kaoutar said in our conversation:

> I will talk to them. I will ask them if they want to become pregnant right now. If they say no then I will talk to them about contraception. I will ask if they are using one. If they are not, then I will tell them about the birth control pill or the IUD. The other methods are not popular. It is important that they use one if they do not want a child. I tell them that.

After Fatima and Kaoutar stated that they would have this counseling session with female patients after a negative pregnancy test, I anticipated having the opportunity to observe it in the clinics during the remaining months of my fieldwork in Rabat. After speaking with Fatima and Kaoutar on different occasions about this, I expected to regularly observe this discussion about family planning after a negative pregnancy test. However, this conversation rarely ever occurred.

> The first woman was 22 years old and had a baby girl. The little girl looked to be pretty young yet. She was being carried in one of the things that you strap on your body. She was not pregnant at this time and seemed pretty happy about it. The second woman who came in was 28 years old. She said she already had two children, but I don't know if they are girls or boys. She was also not pregnant and had a very positive reaction. Obviously she didn't want to have another child at this moment, but there was not talk of contraception. She was just given the paper and left the room. The two female interns who were in the room with Kaoutar were surprised as to this woman's reactions. They did not expect it. . . . After her came in a 28 year old who wore a bright orange djellaba. She had make up and looked to be very stylish. She had a big smile on her face when she found out she was not pregnant. (Excerpt from field notes March 27, 2008)

When women found out they were expecting, Fatima and Kaoutar would ask if they were planning to come back to see an OB/GYN at the clinic for an ultrasound and checkup. Women who were not pregnant did not receive any sort of in-depth counseling at the time of their negative result. In speaking with Dr. Mohammed, a director at the Ministry of Health, about this, she stated, "Yes, I know. We have problems. This needs to be taken care of. We have big problems in Morocco." What happened instead was a conversation that revolved more so around women's beliefs in God and their religious understandings than medical recommendations. In other words, discourses about belief intersected with medical discourses in the space of the counseling room.

The absence of this conversation illustrates two main ideas. First, it shows that there are unintended results of medical intervention, and in fact it demonstrates that technologies like the pregnancy test are not forms of pure intervention but rather methods for the production of new religious identities and new ideas about what it means to be modern. Second, this absence highlights that the medical is not completely replaced or offset by belief or by religion, but rather it is morphed into something new that combines all of these. This is not particularly what the government and RHO had intended, but in the end the results are the same. There are large-scale campaigns in Morocco to bring women into the clinics for reproductive healthcare in part because maternal mortality in the country remains higher than desired by the government and public health community, but the reasoning behind these efforts rely upon women realizing that medical technologies will only improve their health—having a rapid pregnancy test will encourage women to either seek maternal healthcare immediately or to seek other medical attention if they are trying to become pregnant but cannot. But the female patients I observed did not follow this particular logic. Instead they saw the test as a possible work of God because God will control whether it is positive or negative and in addition as a way to improve themselves as Muslims. They will be able to better care for their smaller number of children when a test is negative.

The relationship between believing and acting voluntarily is contested in anthropology. I am not specifically interested in distilling the status of Moroccan women's belief in God in relation to their knowledge nor am I contending that believing and acting are mutually exclusive. In drawing on the formulation of Thomas Kirsch (2004), I suggest discourses about belief and ways of believing are put into practice through pregnancy tests in the clinics. Belief in God is essential to Moroccan women's religious practices, but there is a distinction here between belief in God and Islam; one does not mean the other (Bruce 1992; Haring 1973). Female patients who expressed their joy at discovering they were not pregnant believed that God had helped them become better Muslims, mothers, and citizens by ensuring that their tests were negative. This allowed them to put key Islamic tenets concerning fertility and motherhood into practice, which in reality overlap the rhetoric of responsibility promoted by the INDH. This further demonstrates that the modern citizen in Morocco is produced in part through popular understandings of Islam. On this note, I reiterate that the relationship between religion and medical technologies is highly complex. Inhorn (2004) and Sargent (2006) have masterfully demonstrated that Islamic beliefs and practices impact men and women's reproductive decision making in the Middle East and the diaspora, but such scholars assume that this relationship is one-sided. My female participants suggested to me that reproductive technologies actually inform how they "believe" in God and what they believe that Islam says about fertility, pregnancy, and mothering.

Female patients negotiated believing in the scientific aspects of the pregnancy test (allowing them to know whether or not they were pregnant within just a few minutes) with their beliefs in God's will. Women often called upon God after they received their desired or undesired results, which meant that the biological and scientific were not separate from their religious beliefs. In observing women's reactions, I noted that medical reasoning (i.e., conception either did or did not take place due to the nonuse or use of contraception) was not granted more authority than God or religion. The pregnancy test becomes a way for women to make "belief statements" and to live out what they understand Islam to say about fertility and motherhood.

## "I CAN'T, GOD KNOWS IT": THE ECONOMIC AND PHYSICAL HARDSHIPS OF CHILDBEARING AND CHILDREARING

One morning I sat in the counseling room at Tarma with Habiba. She was the cleaning lady at the RHO clinic a few days a week. Habiba had four children, two boys and two girls, who were all grown. Two of them lived in the local area and two lived farther away. At the time of my fieldwork, Habiba was in her early fifties. Every day that I saw her at the clinic she was dressed in white clothes and a matching hijab. Fatima and Habiba were coworkers and friends, and Habiba often joined Fatima and me when we ate lunch together. Often Habiba would give women advice in the waiting or counseling rooms and would help Fatima with small tasks around the clinic. On this occasion I was observing patients and Habiba was taking a quick break from her duties. Having her in the counseling room with us made it extremely cramped as it was not a large room to begin with, but patients still came in one by one to be checked in by Fatima.

A woman had come into the counseling room this day in her midthirties. She came for a pregnancy test and was prepared with a jar of urine that she had collected that morning. Fatima took a drop of urine and placed it on the stick. She told the woman to wait outside until her name was called. She did so and sat on a chair not too far away from the door. You could see her peering in every few minutes to see if Fatima had looked at her test yet. A few minutes later Fatima called the woman back into the room for her result. She was not pregnant, but I missed the complete exchange between her and Fatima due to another woman coming into the room and briefly talking to me. I asked Habiba what happened. Our conversation went like this:

| | |
|---|---|
| *CORTNEY:* | She isn't pregnant? |
| *HABIBA:* | No, she's not pregnant. |
| *CORTNEY:* | She's happy, no? |
| *HABIBA:* | Yes, she's very happy. God understands. She has two children now and three is too many (*bzzaf*). |

Like this woman, the majority of female patients I observed were thrilled to hear the news that they were not pregnant. Whereas this woman was excited that she was not expecting her third child, Habiba explained her joy with a reference to what God understood about her life. This woman, as were the majority of patients, was working class, and perhaps she could not afford more than just a few children. The medical community in Morocco describes two children as being "perfect" (*parfait*) and three as being "not bad" (*pas grave*). Habiba did not draw on such public health discourses about reproduction to justify the woman's reactions, but rather she emphasized what God knew about the woman's circumstances. God would not give her more than she, her body, and her family could handle.

Women's responses to their pregnancy tests often combined their religious beliefs with economic constraints. One woman who discovered she was not pregnant told Fatima outright after receiving her results, "I can't. God knows it." Fatima explained that many women do not want to have another child because their bodies become too tired and they are exhausted from all the work involved, but also raising children can be expensive. What I want to point out here is that the practical reasoning for not wanting to have another child, the fact that giving birth and caring for a baby is tiresome, and the financial reasoning, children cost money, were couched within women's beliefs in God. This reshapes the relationship between belief and action and between medical and religious discourses. Lock et al. argue that medical technologies cannot be theorized as "things-in-themselves" (2000, 12) nor can they be thought of as separate from the body or the social, political, and historical contexts in which the body is conceived. Taking up this claim, I point out that pregnancy tests are highly entangled within Moroccan women's beliefs in God and within their Islamic interpretations of what it means to be a "good" mother.

Of the women I informally interviewed, about half made direct mention of the work they must do around their homes during our conversations. This was in fact a major concern of the female patients as well as the medical providers. Patients who did work as housekeepers or in the local markets often did so up until just a few days before they delivered and then they returned to work just a couple of weeks after giving birth. Foreign friends of mine who shared an apartment in Rabat had a Moroccan housekeeper who worked up until she was eight and a half months pregnant. They asked her at about six months to take some time off to rest and prepare for her new arrival, but she refused because she already had three young boys to support financially, one who had learning and physical disabilities due to a bad fall when he was a toddler, and another little boy on the way. After the birth of her most recent child, she would have four mouths to feed and needed the money to do so. Even at eight and a half months along, it was a struggle for them to get her to quit working at their apartment because they were afraid she would go into labor early. (She eventually allowed her sister to take over cleaning and went on to have a healthy baby boy a few days after her official due date.) Those women who worked only within their own homes typically had a short period of time after birth before they needed to get back to cleaning, cooking, and doing the laundry. Both groups of women, those who held employment outside the home and those who did not, typically did not have a long enough time to rest and prepare prior to going into labor or to recover from their pregnancies and births. After negative pregnancy tests, several female patients at the RHO's clinics expressed concern that they physically, emotionally, and financially could not take care of a child. In particular, many women made reference to their own bodies and expressed that they could not handle the stress of childbearing and childrearing. If they were not taking care of themselves, then they could not possibly give children all of the support and attention they need to develop into the healthy, productive, and responsible citizens Morocco desires.

## DISCOVERING PREGNANCY: REACTING TO POSITIVE PREGNANCY TESTS

> I was looking through my fieldnotes today from the clinics. I took note of something that I hadn't particularly noticed before when I was actually jotting them down in the counseling room. When I went back through my notes I kept seeing the word "unhappy" or the phrase "not happy" scribbled over various pages. I looked at each of the cases in which I had written this word or phrase and in each one it was in reference to a pregnancy test. The women didn't have negative pregnancy tests, but rather positive pregnancy tests. They were disappointed that they were expecting, some of them for the first time and some for the third or fourth time. Most women who were pregnant for the second time did not seem to be too distraught unless they felt they did not have enough space between their children. (Excerpt from field notes June 25, 2008)

The majority of women that I observed were thrilled to hear the news they were not pregnant, and, at the same time, several women who found out they were pregnant were very disappointed with their results. One woman, after learning that she was expecting her third child, asked Kaoutar, "*Ana ḥamla*?" or "I'm pregnant?" three times before leaving the clinic. She wanted to make sure that Kaoutar had accurately read her results. Whereas having three children is considered to be acceptable by the medical community in Morocco, and if they are spaced properly three children is looked upon even more favorably, it was obviously not tolerable for this particular patient. I even observed some women physically break down in tears when they heard their test was in fact positive.

> A woman came in for a pregnancy test. She was carrying a small infant with her in a carrier and was 26 years old. After a few minutes Hannen [a substitute for Fatima] called her back in the room to read the results of her test; they were positive. At first she said, "Me?" and then smiled, but then gave a very dissatisfied look. She shriveled her nose a bit and looked to the ground. She pointed out that her baby is very young yet and it isn't a good time to have another child. A 36-year-old woman came in the room for a pregnancy test. Before knowing the results Hannen told her that if she is pregnant she needs to return for a sonogram. She wore glasses, with a long skirt, and loose blouse. Hannen gave her the paper, which stated her test results were positive. She stared at the paper for a long time while hunched over the desk, then she asked, "But why God?" Hannen told her about the pill and the IUD because it was obvious she did not want to have a child. After she left the room I asked Hannen why women don't use contraception if they don't want to have children. She just smiled and shrugged her shoulders without ever responding to the question. (Excerpt from field notes June 4, 2008)

One morning at the Tarma clinic, two women came into the counseling room. The one woman was there for the pregnancy test and the other was her sister. The sister did all of the talking to Fatima and the patient barely said a word. They were both dressed in black djellabas and matching colored hijabs. The patient did manage to tell Fatima her age, twenty-six, and place of residence, a working-class neighborhood near the clinic. Just by looking at the female patient you could tell she was very anxious about having the test. She was quiet but could not stand still while in the counseling room. She was so nervous she was almost shaking. Her petite body was engulfed by her oversize black djellaba. Fatima took a sample of urine from the jar she brought with her and placed it on the testing stick, the standard procedure. The two women exited the room and sat down in the waiting room. I could see them looking at the door. Fatima called them in a few minutes later when the results were ready. The young woman was pregnant with her third child. Fatima told her this and her sister immediately responded, "*B-sah! Hiya ḥ'mla?*" ("Really! She's pregnant?") in amazement. The sister turned to the patient to tell her that she was indeed expecting. The patient immediately broke down. She sat in the chair in the counseling room and began to cry. She wiped away her tears with the sleeves of her djellaba and the corners of her hijab. She rocked back and forth. I managed to find a tissue in my bag and offered it to her, which she accepted with a slight smile through her tears. Fatima inquired if she would return to see the doctor at the clinic for an ultrasound and consultation within the next few weeks. The sister explained that after two children, her doctor had told the patient that she should not become pregnant again because she has a very small uterus. Another pregnancy could cause major damage to her uterus or it could even rupture, possibly causing death due to internal bleeding. The sister did not mention if the doctor had discussed using contraception with her or not. The two women left the counseling room and, as they did, the sister said they would return soon for a follow-up visit with the doctor.

After the sisters left, Fatima explained that this woman was very sad because her husband did not care about her health. She made a gesture with her hand when she said this, flicking her wrist like she was dusting something off her desk. The woman's husband wanted another child immediately, according to the sister, and so she became pregnant again. Fatima said, "Her husband wants another baby now so she became pregnant. She's very sad. She already has two children. She's so little! I don't think she went to school so she does not have her own money, she does not work, but she is very scared her husband will leave her if she did not become pregnant again. So she did. *C'est dommage* [It's a shame/pity]." Fatima was very critical of this patient's husband and was less than pleased that he had put pressure on her to have another baby given her condition. Fatima then went on to say, "I don't understand. He isn't a Muslim. Why? Why does he want her to be pregnant again? She has problems. God doesn't want this." Even though children are considered gifts from God for Muslims and the number of children one has is determined by God (Libbus and Kridli 2002), verses from the Qur'an emphasize that God does not wish to create undue stress for anyone (Franzmann 2010). For instance, the Qur'an reads:

> The Apostle believes in what has been revealed to him by his Lord, and so do the faithful. They all believe in God and His angels, His scriptures, and His apostles. We discriminate against none of His apostles. They say: "We hear and obey. Grant us Your forgiveness, Lord; to You shall all return. God does not charge a soul with more than it can bear. it shall be requited for whatever good and whatever evil it has done. Lord, do not be angry with us if we forget or lapse into error. Lord, do not lay on us a burden such as You laid on those before us. Lord, do not charge us with more than we can bear. Pardon us, forgive us our sins, and have mercy upon us. You alone are our Protector. Give us victory over the unbelievers." (2:285–286)

Fatima assumed that this man did not take care of his wife properly, as Islam states a man should, because he did not respect her health. In her opinion, he was not deemed as a proper Muslim because he wanted another child and neglected his wife's physical condition. His wife's sister confided in Fatima that she was scared he would leave her if she did not fulfill his wishes and try to become pregnant again. However, as the previous verse shows, Islam does not intend for people to be burdened financially or physically, leading to the conclusion that quality of children is much more important than quantity (Keefe 2006). For Fatima, there is a very clear distinction between a proper Muslim and one who is not. The patient's husband did not follow the "correct understanding" of Islam when it came to his wife and his family.[5]

Some women at the health clinics who took pregnancy tests were excited to discover they were expecting a child. One woman in her late thirties who had been following infertility treatments with one of the doctors at the Tarma clinic was overjoyed to find out that she was pregnant with her first child. After a few years of following such treatments with the doctor and Fatima, her wish had finally come true. After Fatima read the test results, she even asked her if she could wrap up her positive test so that she could show her husband later at home. Fatima obliged and hugged and kissed the woman before she left the counseling room. She wished her luck and reminded her to come back in a few weeks for an ultrasound and checkup. However, this woman's reaction was far from the norm over the course of my fieldwork, and I rarely saw another woman exhibit such joy even when she was happy to be pregnant.

Fatima also leveled critiques after a woman came in for an ultrasound one afternoon. The patient was three months pregnant at the time, and Fatima said she had taken a pregnancy test at the clinic about two months prior. This was her follow-up visit and the first time seeing the doctor since discovering she was expecting her second child. She already had a son, who was eight months old. When women return to the clinic for a follow-up, they are required to go up the street in Tarma for blood work at a local laboratory. Blood tests are routine at the beginning of each pregnancy. The clinic in Zitounia has a technician from a local laboratory collect the samples a few days a week, but the one in Tarma does not have someone to do this. So women will need to travel about a mile (1.6 kilometers) to the center of Tarma to a laboratory that works with the RHO. The blood tests are used to measure basic levels, such as cholesterol and particular nutrients like iron. I asked Fatima how it could be possible for this woman to become pregnant while breastfeeding her son, as it is recommended to do for two years. Fatima explained that this woman's husband had made her wean the boy early so that he could have another child close in age to his son. He did not want too much time in between his children, and, therefore, his wife became pregnant again within a very short time after giving birth even though it could be detrimental to her health and the well-being of their children.

Fatima was very disappointed with this patient's husband and with the patient for complying with his wishes even though it could put her body at risk given there was little time in between her pregnancies. Mrs. Fisher, a feminist activist and American staff member at a university in Morocco, stated that under the revised personal status code (*Moudawana*) husbands cannot divorce their wives if they do not or cannot have children without the consent of a judge. Being infertile (or refusing to become pregnant at a particular time) is not legal grounds for divorce.[6] However, the foregoing patients' stories from the Tarma clinic suggest there is still fear among women that they will be divorced if they do not become pregnant when their husbands want them to do so. Fatima wondered why the patient's husband would be so adamant that he had to have another child right away if he correctly understood what Islam says about reproduction and breastfeeding. Again, the verse from the Qur'an states, with a slightly different translation, "Mothers shall give suck to their children for two whole years if the father wishes the sucking to be completed. They must be maintained and clothed in a reasonable manner by the child's father. None should be charged with more than one can bear. A mother should not be allowed to suffer on account of her child, nor should a father on account of his child" (2:233). The Qur'an suggests that when breastfeeding occurs, it should be done for an extended period of time. Fatima was convinced that this man was not a true Muslim because he gave his wife no option but to have another child so soon. To her, it was obvious that he did not understand the "correct meaning" of Islam (Deeb 2006). Even though Fatima was upset with the woman, questioning her about why she became pregnant just a few months after giving birth, greater anger was expressed at her husband for exerting control over his wife and her health.

This critique of a person's status as a Muslim was mixed with concerns over whether or not a family could financially and physically handle a single or additional child at the time. In conversations with patients about their pregnancy tests, clinical staff deployed a process of "authentication," a concept put forth by Lara Deeb (2006) in her work on gender in Shi'i Lebanon. She describes "authentication" as based upon "a process of establishing true or correct meaning, understanding or method of various religious and social practices" (2006, 20). For example, one of the interns named Farah, who was studying to become a midwife, stated one morning with dismay when a sixteen-year-old came in for her follow-up ultrasound after a positive test, "That is not Islam. She's a little girl!" References to God surfaced again and again in women's reactions to their tests because they believed that God knew as well as compensated them for their poorer economic and social circumstances; however, the clinical staff held specific understandings as to what being a "good" Muslim meant in regards to childbearing and childrearing based upon their readings of the sacred texts and their interpretations.[7] I noticed that the clinical staff members were often more critical of the reproductive desires and practices of women's male counterparts claiming, as Fatima did so often, that they did not know "true" Islam.

## CONCLUSION

Zsuzsa Berend writes in her work on miscarriages among surrogate mothers, "Pregnancy is understood in ways that transcend medical technology" (2010, 245). Berend argues that pregnancy has come to be thought of as a "purposeful undertaking over which [women] have control; medical advice tells them how to take care of themselves to have healthy babies . . . not having control over childbearing, to be sure, calls into question profound . . . assumptions about agency and goal-oriented behavior" (ibid.). Female patients who visited the RHO's clinics in Rabat were provided the information and services they needed in order to make the best decisions about their reproductive practices. Medical staff encouraged them to be "goal-oriented" and to make informed choices about childbearing that would improve their well-being and that of their families and of the nation. However, what is striking in their joyful reactions to negative pregnancy tests is that they relinquished control over their bodies, the process of conception, and the test results. They instead placed their fate and the future of their family into God's hands, not displacing the scientific facts, but rather bringing them together with their religious beliefs. This became clearer to me when so many female patients thanked God for the negative test results or questioned His will when they discovered they were indeed expecting.

This chapter delved into the complex matrices of meanings that surround rapid pregnancy tests in Morocco (Boddy 1989). The pregnancy test is far from a modern medical invention, but rather it takes on many different connotations. Feminist scholars have argued that sonograms inhabit the "private imaginary" of women because they provide a glimpse inside the womb and of their unborn child (Sandelowski 1993). Similarly, the rapid pregnancy test can be a visualizing technology because it enables women to see whether or not they are pregnant within just a few minutes, right after the one line or two lines appear, and gives them a vague picture of their realities and futures as women and mothers. In the health clinics, Moroccan women interpreted the pregnancy test in ways that differed from but yet intersected with the medical professionals, in particular Fatima and Kaoutar. This reproductive technology is not located purely within the scientific realm as is commonly thought, but it can be found at the interstices of circulating discourses of medicine, religion, and belief. Pregnancy tests can help us rethink humans' relationships to medical technologies and the work that such technologies do on the body, mind, and soul. Whereas this chapter has focused on how the "positive on a . . . pregnancy test is . . . construed as indicative of the beginning of life" (Berend 2010, 245), the next chapter focuses on childrearing and motherhood. It takes a critical look at what women understand the model future Moroccan citizen to be and what they need to do as mothers in order to produce such an individual.

# 6 Raising the Next Generation of Moroccan Citizens to Have "Good Hearts"

One afternoon the waiting area of the RHO clinic in Zitounia was crowded with women. They filled the chairs that lined the walls of the room. A very active little boy named Anas was running around. His mother, a woman in her late twenties, was having trouble keeping him under control. She appeared very frustrated and eventually just ignored his rowdy behavior, which was obviously disturbing the other women as they waited patiently to see the doctor. A second young woman accompanied Anas's mother to the clinic that day. She was her cousin who was visiting her from a city in southern Morocco. While Anas's mother was in the exam room, the boy hit her cousin on the head so hard that tears came to her eyes. She put her head in her hands and started to cry. The other women in the waiting room, who were left to watch Anas while his mother was away, scolded him and told his mother as soon as she returned. Anas was physically scared of his mother's reaction and cowered in fear behind one of the chairs. She was extremely displeased with his behavior and began to yell, drawing attention to the situation.

Two other women in the waiting room asked Anas's mother why he was not in school that day. She said that he did not want to learn, and he begged her to stay home. Anas was her and her husband's only child at the time. She eventually agreed to his request because her husband worked outside of the home. The two women shook their heads in dismay. The one woman, Ghizlane, asked the mother, "How is he to learn? What will he learn in the home with you? There is nothing there." The other women in the waiting room joined the inquisition. Anas's mother was not in disagreement with Ghizlane nor was she apologetic for her decision to allow him to miss class. She just explained that it was difficult to raise a young boy and sometimes she had to give in to what he wanted. Ghizlane stated that she understood her situation because she had three young children at home, but children's desires to play are no reason to keep them from going to school. Ghizlane acknowledged that the public school system in Morocco has many flaws, but she claimed that children are able to learn more there than they could if they stayed at home with their mothers: "I can teach my children to cook and clean. What does that do?"

This type of conversation occurred again and again in the waiting rooms of the RHO clinics in Tarma and Zitounia. Inadvertently I would join discussions about what it means to be a "good" mother that were taking place in the rooms or in the sewing classes offered to the women in Tarma, which I sat in on from time to time. One woman in the class mentioned as she was sewing a pair of pants, "I sell these clothes for my children." These conversations about motherhood were usually trans-generational, involving older women giving younger women advice, or they involved more experienced mothers, like Ghizlane, who was raising more than one child, and those less experienced, similar to Anas's mother, who had only one child or were expecting. And, of course, these discussions also involved women who had yet to conceive, like myself. These conversations demonstrate motherhood is truly a dynamic and culturally informed process that involves several individuals and changes given the economic, social, and political climate of the time and place. The individuals involved in the discussions were not always related to each other through blood or marriage. Therefore, the waiting rooms became spaces where relations between women were reconstructed. In the many conversations that I observed over the course of my fieldwork, the women were strangers who had met each other for the first time when they came to the same clinic seeking reproductive healthcare. Motherhood was a point of agreement as well as debate. The waiting areas, in addition to the sewing classroom, offered women spaces where they could share their frustrations, excitements, fears, methods, and definitions of "good" motherhood.

Silence is a critical theme that runs throughout scholarship on feminine citizenship and identities in the MENA (Lazreg 1994; Schaefer-Davis 1983). Mernissi (1988) argues the silence of women is one of the foundations upon which Moroccan society is built. The Morocco produced through women's eyes differs from that which is described through popular culture, legislation, development policies, and national politics. Problems and struggles are cast in a new light. Mernissi writes of Morocco, "The world that emerges through the words of women is a world fundamentally different from the world prescribed as ideal by the 'pervasive' male discourse" (1988, 4). However, I argue the silence Mernissi details is eradicated inside the clinics' waiting rooms and the sewing classroom as Moroccan women bring together various scales and temporalities as well as personal experiences in order to grapple with the meanings of "good" motherhood being produced at the present moment. Rapid transformations in healthcare and new development discourses help obliterate this silence as they make negotiating new definitions and practices of motherhood an absolute must. The waiting room was a contested space where the private affairs of the family and women's bodies converged with medical practices, health discourses, and larger ideas about motherhood. Female patients were the authorities in this space, but their authority was relinquished once they were with the medical staff in private.[1]

With posters lining the walls advocating methods of contraception and techniques of mothering, the clinic is constructed as a site of intervention by the state and the RHO. However, this space was also where the values associated with being a mother, definitions of motherhood, and the attributes of the "desired child" were reconfigured on a daily basis. Women are producing something new—new ways of mothering, new ways of addressing politics, and new ways of raising future citizens. Women continue to work within this domain of intervention, but they transform it at the same time. The clinic was a space where power is dispersed (Foucault 1994). The state and the RHO conduct surveillance of the female patients by intervening in their most intimate human affairs: fertility and health (Farquhar and Zhang 2005; Foucault 1994). However, the Moroccan women who visited the clinic used the waiting room for their own purposes as well. Rather than being a place of strict acceptance of government ideologies and medical practices, I argue, the interactions in the waiting room and sewing classroom fostered new notions of feminine identity through the reconfiguration of relationships between women. Women, like Anas's mother and Ghizlane in Zitounia, stopped being strangers to one another and built new relationships as they strived for change together.

Scholars have defined the "good" mother in many different ways. Donald Winnicott (1965), for example, draws on psychoanalysis in his formulation of the "good enough mother," or a mother who is attentive to her child's needs but sometimes slow to respond. The lag time between when the child expresses the need and the mother's actual response helps the child develop into an independent being. Another theorization comes from Donna Bassin, Margaret Honey, and Merle Mahrer Kaplan (1994). They contend in the dominant motherhood ideology the "good" mother is portrayed as being devoted to the care of others. She is "not a subject with her own needs and interests" (Bassin et al. 1994, 2). Their suggestion and Winnicott's concept both resonate in the constructions of motherhood that women in Morocco read or see every day. Within the context of the INDH, mothers are supposed to create independent citizens who will not rely upon the state for assistance. They are to do so, however, through caring for and nurturing their children.

This chapter examines the novel ideas of modern motherhood that come out of conversations in the waiting rooms of the clinics and traces how these definitions are put into practice in everyday life. Whereas childbearing is of great importance to the creation of modern Morocco, childrearing is also given tremendous weight as women are expected to instill certain qualities into the future citizens they are raising. For the mothers I worked with, in order to be modern and successful in the future, children need to be taught how to live a prosperous and economically viable life, but, at the same time, they must be taught how to be moral and how to further their faith and religious knowledge. What this chapter shows is that material wealth is not separate from religious growth for the women and mothers that I observed and interviewed. What I ultimately demonstrate is that childrearing is just one more way that Moroccan working-class women have appropriated the neoliberal rhetoric of development that comes with the INDH. Through their conversations in the waiting rooms and through their childrearing practices, women have created new meanings of good motherhood and new expectations of the future modern child.

## WAITING, WAITING, WAITING

Women spend a great deal of time in the waiting rooms, much more so than they spend with the doctor in the exam rooms. Sometimes women would arrive as early only to be seen in the afternoon, around noon or 1:00 p.m., when the doctor finally arrived. Some would come and go, others would sit and wait, some would watch television, and some would sleep. But most often, women made conversation with one another. On one occasion six women lined the wall of the Tarma waiting room just outside of the sewing classroom. They ranged in age, and two of these women had brought their toddlers with them. The one little boy was extremely active and was no more than three years old. He ran around the waiting room, whereas the little girl stayed close to her mother. The boy's mother would run after him again and again as he darted out the main entrance. She spanked him numerous times, and he would cry before running around again. The other women yelled at her when she did this, asking her why, but she would just yell back at them in frustration. She did not know another way to get him to listen to her other than physical force. She gestured wildly with her hands as she defended her mothering techniques.

Another woman brought her daughter with her when she participated in the sewing class. The little girl, named Dahlia, was only three years old and would busily pretend to sew as her mother actually made various garments. All of the women in the sewing class would dote on Dahlia, asking her to bring them supplies or hold fabric. Dahlia's mother, who had no other children at the time, explained that she wanted her daughter to sew in the future with her, but only after she gained an education. School was most important and sewing came second. When Dahlia's mother explained this the other women in the classroom agreed with her thinking and emphasized school was absolutely *moheem* (necessary) for her daughter. Whereas the young boy's mother was scolded for her mothering practices, Dahlia's mother was congratulated and supported by the other women in the sewing room. The waiting room (in addition to the sewing classroom) was one of the most important places where women learned about the cultural constructions and norms of motherhood through receiving advice, being scolded or encouraged by other women, or engaging in small debates. The relationship between non-kin women was transformed while they inhabited these spaces as mothers (or future mothers). I describe these areas as contested because women are the authorities of childbearing and childrearing in them, not the medical staff (Davis-Floyd and Sargent 1997). The patients and friends and family who accompanied them draw on medical, development, social, and religious discourses in their own ways to educate one another.

In the health clinics, medical providers, posters and pamphlets, and daily conversations attempted to foster a mentality in patients that was conducive to the acceptance of modern contraceptive methods, prenatal care, and "good" mothering practices, such as breastfeeding. The clinic operates through ideology and discourse rather than repression (Althusser 1971). This is evident through the staff's claims that they are not allowed to force a woman to use any of the services. They can only make recommendations; however, sometimes women are given a very limited number of choices that will only result in their acceptance of a particular service.

Women themselves actively engage in the education of other patients within particular spaces (El Shakry 2007). Moroccan women have learned what it means to be "good" mothers through several different mediums, some of which are based on self-education whereas others are more directed and not so subtle. The ultimate recipients of the benefits from women engaging in practices of "good" motherhood are their children. Two particular educational methods stood out to me on a regular basis during my fieldwork: conversations between the counselors and patients and informal conversations that took place in female patients' homes.

## SELF-RECOGNITION AND ADVICE GIVING: SHAME AND BLAME DURING COUNSELING SESSIONS

Proper mothering practices were promoted not only through conversations in the waiting rooms, but also during the counseling sessions. Discussions of good childrearing practices were common between the female patients and the counselors, Fatima and Kaoutar. One Thursday morning in Zitounia, Kaoutar checked in women who came to see the OB/GYN on staff that day, Dr. Senah. One older woman came into the room. She wanted a consultation with the doctor. Kaoutar asked the basic questions that counselors posed to all first-time patients, which included inquiring about how many children the women already have and how many they would like to have total. This particular woman responded that she had four children and she does not want any more. She had two boys and two girls. As Kaoutar was writing this information in her chart, the woman offered, "I know. This is a lot." Kaoutar looked up and said, "No, not a lot" in a comforting manner, even though counselors and doctors recommend a woman have no more than three children.

Next, Kaoutar asked this woman, "Do they all study? Do the girls?" The woman, who had since taken a seat near Kaoutar's desk, nodded her head in agreement. She then stated that all of her children attended or are still attending school. Some of her children who were old enough were working and living elsewhere outside of their natal home. Kaoutar responded that children's education is extremely important and that she was happy this mother managed to send all of her children to school because some Moroccan women are not able to do so. Like Ghizlane's comments, discussed in the beginning of this chapter, Kaoutar's focus was on the need for children to be educated in a public institution—somewhere other than the home. She explained to this woman that educating girls and boys is necessary in order for them to understand that they must in turn educate their own children in the future. Fatima, Dr. Senah, Dr. Mamouri, Dr. Mohammed, and executive staff at the RHO emphasized the importance of this cycle also. However, rather quickly, Kaoutar and this patient's conversation shifted directions as Kaoutar reminded her that according to Islam and to God, the education of mothers and future mothers is not optional (*xṣṣhm ydrsu* ) but is a must because it will only improve the lives of their children.

Moroccan women recognized the societal norms associated with children, such as educating young girls, and when these norms were violated, women often expressed their shame to the counselors. They shamed themselves when they realized that they had stepped outside of the boundaries set by the government, medical community, and their fellow Moroccan citizens. In observing the counseling sessions at the RHO clinics, I took note that women who had two or three children would state this matter-of-factly to Fatima or Kaoutar. Women would take pride in this accomplishment, which resonated in their speech and how they carried themselves. However, on several occasions, women who had more than the recommended number of children would feel the need to justify this to the counselor. This includes the woman mentioned earlier who stated, "I know. This is a lot." (*Knarf. Hada bzzaf.*) At times, women would physically react to the disappointment that they knew would soon come from Fatima or Kaoutar, who would also give women a mini-lecture from time to time of the importance of regulating fertility. This is illustrated in a short excerpt taken from my field notes from the Tarma clinic.

> Next, an older woman came into the counseling room and sat in the chair near the window. Fatima remained seated behind her desk as this woman made her way across the small room to sit down. She wore a light blue [hijab] and a darker blue djellaba. She appeared to be in her fifties and was slightly heavy set. A few brownish gray hairs were noticeable from under her [hijab]. She leaned on the desk with her one elbow as Fatima asked her the basic questions. She had come in for a consultation with the OB/GYN . . . Fatima then asked her how many children she had [*shal?*] but the woman looked down to the floor. She kept her head propped up on her one hand and then started to play with the fabric of her djellaba with the other. She almost appeared to be

> a little nervous and uncomfortable. She mumbled *khmsa* [five]. Fatima didn't hear her at first. I did because I was sitting in the chair next to the wall and I was only a foot away or so. Fatima asked again *shal*? The woman again responded *khmsa*, but this time just slightly louder. This woman looked sad. It was almost like she knew that Fatima would not be happy with her. (Excerpt from field notes June 9, 2008)

The woman's inability to sit still, her locked stare at the floor, and her barely audible words indicated that she understood the number of children she had exceeded the state and medical community's recommendations. When women stated they had five or six (or sometimes more) children, Fatima and Kaoutar would often ask why they had so many. Women usually did not have an answer to this question; they just responded, "I don't know" or shrugged their shoulders.

Having a larger number of children should raise concern for working-class women according to the staff at the health clinics, the state, and development agencies. They should be worried about educating their children and about whether or not their children's bodies can be cared for physically. I observed this type of self-recognition and self-shaming over the course of my fieldwork. Female patients who had several children or who were young in age, mostly teenagers, would become physically uncomfortable when discussing their situations with the counselors. On one occasion an older woman escorted a sixteen-year-old into the clinic for her first ultrasound. She was married and was expecting her first child. The woman spoke softly to Fatima as if she did not want anyone else to hear that the pregnant woman, who was her daughter, was still a teenager. The woman gripped the teenager's hand tightly during the in-take interview and would not allow her to speak even though Fatima addressed her directly. Moroccan women were well aware of the norms the counselors expected them to follow regarding their childbearing and childrearing. As demonstrated above, a number of women expressed disappointment when they did not conform to these standards and ideals of "good" motherhood; others acted joyful and proud when they knew that they adhered to these guidelines.

## TALKING ABOUT MODERNITY AND DEFINING "GOOD" MOTHERHOOD

When women become mothers they must negotiate the various kinds of information they receive that details what exactly it means to be a "good" mother (Paxson 2004; Wall 2001). Many sources intersected with Islamic discourses of responsibility and how to be accountable to the family and the larger community through particular mothering practices that are based upon religious beliefs and tenets. This creates an entirely new set of ethics and new questions about what it means to be a responsible mother.

Often women spoke about development in reference to their children's futures rather than in terms of their own lives. It was not so much about their fate, even though this was important, but rather about how they were going to help their children succeed in the future through adopting specific childrearing practices at the present. Some women even expressed fear about becoming mothers, which I suggest represents the possibility that they may not be able to help their children fulfill their societal roles and expectations due to constraining life circumstances. Amina's story illustrates this point. Amina was twenty-eight years old when she came with her sister to the RHO clinic in Tarma to see the gynecologist. Her sister was there for a follow-up visit for her IUD and was very nervous, so Amina came with her that day. Amina was training to become a nurse and she wanted to practice in France when she graduated from nursing school because her husband was already living there. He is Moroccan by descent, but is a French citizen. He lived outside of Paris most of the year, but would return to Morocco every few months to visit Amina. After she completed her studies, Amina planned to move to France full-time and to look for employment in the nursing field. By the time my fieldwork was coming to a close in the summer of 2009, Amina had fulfilled her goal of living in France, but she had yet to find a job as a nurse.

Amina and her husband did not have any children. When I asked her if they wanted children, she responded inshallah that they will have two or three in the future once they are settled in France. Amina said she wanted to wait until she lived in France before they even started trying to conceive. I asked if the reason why she wanted to wait was because she wanted her children to grow up with both their mother and father in the same household. She responded that this was part of the reason. A second issue was that she wanted her husband to quit smoking before they had children because it is not good for his health and could be detrimental to her health as well as that of their children. However, the main reason Amina gave me as to why she was delaying pregnancy was that she does not want to give birth or raise her children in Morocco. She made it seem as though this was a mutual agreement between her and her husband. Amina stated she felt that life was too hard in Morocco for boys and girls, and it was equally difficult for parents to raise children is such an environment where there are fewer job opportunities and the education system has been highly criticized by parents, activists, and scholars. Amina described the future as *sombre* or bleak. She was convinced that her children's lives, her own, and her husband's would be much better if they lived in France than in Morocco.

Amina was cautious about becoming pregnant. Her fear about pregnancy highlights her concerns about her family's future in Morocco. This fear also illustrates the discrepancies between the future that she wants for her children and what is expected of her as a modern mother, and the actual future she believes her children will have if she chooses to stay in Morocco and raise them in the country. Amina would not be able to reach the societal expectations for motherhood—educating her children and providing them opportunities to grow personally and academically—if she remained in Morocco while raising them. Amina showed great concern about the number and quality of educational and professional possibilities that will be open to her children as they become older. I see Amina's story as a metaphor for the larger and more complex political and economic shifts that have occurred in Morocco in the recent decades, specifically those revolving around the effect of global market integration and the restructuring of education. These shifts have helped shape modern notions of what is considered to be responsible motherhood. Amina intended to delay becoming a mother until she was certain she could fulfill this role by guaranteeing that her children receive a good education and a broader range of job opportunities in the future. This can only take place in France, not Morocco according to her.

For Amina, being a responsible mother was hinged upon the guarantee that she will be able to provide a life that is not so *sombre* for her children, even if it means moving to Europe in order to do so. What is striking here is that Amina's idea of good motherhood actually rests upon the assumption that she must move her family out of Morocco so they can have a larger number of opportunities and maximize their potential as human beings; however, she is doing this so that she can fulfill the expectations associated with responsible citizenship and mothering that exist within Morocco. Interactions and contestations among discourses of development, motherhood, medicine, and gender have a profound impact on how women thought of and described themselves as mothers. I found that women in Morocco often translated their "actions into idioms comprehensible to others" (Newcomb 2008, 5) as they defined themselves as good mothers. Newcomb writes that for women in Morocco, "working within the existing structures of power to gain acceptance for something new" (ibid.) is often a necessity. Amina needed to delay pregnancy and to raise her children in Europe in order to meet the standards of responsible motherhood as set by the Moroccan state and society.

## THE MEANING OF MOTHERHOOD

In earlier feminist scholarship, motherhood was debated and sometimes rejected as "compulsory heterosexuality" (Rich 1980). Feminist scholars had critiqued motherhood as being preceived as the physical and social destiny for all women. Amina thinks about the future through her yet-to-be-conceived children and does not deny that she will become a mother one day to two or three children, but it is evident that state modernization rhetoric of responsibility and self-governance has impacted how she thinks about motherhood and what it means for her to be a proper mother to her children. Lois McNay argues, "feminists regard [motherhood] as one of the main supports of patriarchal domination and also one of the strongholds of feminine identity" (1992, 23–24). McNay contends that this illustrates an "alternative feminist approach" to the body, which is seen as being located at the "threshold of subjectivity." Motherhood is not purely a fixed biological essence nor is it a consequence of social conditioning, but instead it is a combination of both, as Amina's story demonstrates. The reproductive and maternal body is to be theorized as a site where the biological converges with the social and where broader discourses of power merge with women's subjectivities (Barlow 2004; Mabilia 2005). Feminist scholars have argued that it is dangerous to think of the body in just essentialist terms, but it is nearly impossible to deny the corporeal reality of human experience (Casper 1994), including giving birth and raising children.

In this convergence, women produce identities that draw upon the biological essence of motherhood, social constructions of women and mothers, and their conceptions of the future. Approaches to analyzing feminine identities as described by McNay recognize plurality, and I emphasize that new identities are created within this process that actually break down the boundaries between the biological and the social as women negotiate what it means to be "good" mothers in their everyday lives, just as Amina did. Feminist scholars have called attention to the various ways that women deploy concepts of morality and responsibility in regards to motherhood (Ruddick 1989). Carole Gilligan (1982) offers an alternative version of feminine ethics that derives from observations that women's moral judgments are contingent on their relationships with others, particularly their families, and are very contextualized. Morality is based upon caring and relationships as opposed to reason and rationale. This conception of motherhood challenges the devaluation of women's lives and of motherhood. However, at the same time, it only works to construct another universal model of morality, which Gilligan attempts to debunk, and ultimately essentializes women's experiences. There is a strong need to develop a theory of ethics and responsibility surrounding motherhood that takes emotions and relationships into account while not attributing such to women's biological affinity with fertility and childrearing.

However, within the current context of Morocco, this may actually be difficult to do given that I argued state policy and medical practices continue to circumscribe women as mothers for the most part. Whereas the government, medical professionals, and those involved in development attempt to promote a form of liberation and autonomy, there is a constant harking back to the ultimate goal of biological motherhood. Studies of fostering children and of adoption are useful in thinking through this conundrum of how to examine motherhood outside of a biological realm without losing sight of the human body, but in a context where women's ability to give birth and to raise children takes precedence. Emily Walmsley argues that through everyday practices in Ecuador "children become bound" (2008, 169) into the family unit without being related by blood; however, their relationship to their foster parents remains ambiguous. Similarly, Danielle Wozniak (2002) highlights the cultural construction of kinship in America in her in-depth study of foster parents from a variety of socioeconomic statuses. These female foster parents, Wozniak argues, think of kinship in terms of affection that is defined by neither biology nor economic exchange. I fuse together such work by Walmsley and Wozniak with Foucault's (1995) theorization of the body as historically specific and produced through discourse in order to conceptualize how women's reproduction and mothering in Morocco is contextualized within the current political and social climate. Rather than falling back on a notion of biological determinism to analyze motherhood, this section of the chapter interrogates how larger structures of society help frame the ways women discuss their roles as "producers," as mothers, and as citizens. The physical human body does not disappear in my analysis, but rather it is seen as a vehicle for larger forces. I start to illustrate my point by detailing two portraits of mothers in Morocco: Kenza and Layla.

## KENZA: THE REPRODUCTIVE HEALTH ORGANIZATION'S VOLUNTEER

In the summer of 2008, I attended a training session for volunteers who participated in the RHO outreach program. This session took place in Agadir, a large coastal city known for its tourism and beautiful beaches in southern Morocco. Sixteen female volunteers attended the brief two-day training program that was run by Mrs. Asam, a woman who worked for a separate organization that was responsible for providing training to all of the RHO's volunteers in the region. The session took place in a large meeting room at one of the RHO's clinics in Agadir normally used for the clinic's youth group meetings. After the training, the volunteers would return to their towns and villages to disseminate the information that they received and to teach men and women about various aspects of sexual and reproductive health. These trainings ensured that the volunteers received the most up-to-date information about healthcare trends and were knowledgeable about important health issues. All of the women listened intently as she showed slides and offered up-to-date information about STDs, pregnancy, hygienic practices, and common illnesses. Several of the women actively contributed to the discussion about how to improve their skills as volunteers and offered feedback about their experiences "in the field." Over the lunch break, Kenza and I went out onto the balcony to get some fresh air, and we chatted about her work with the RHO. The conversation moved towards her family. At the time she had a son who was six years old and a daughter who was just two years old. Kenza stated:

> My parents promised me to be married when I was just six years old. They did not know anything. When I was sixteen I told them that I didn't want to marry this man. They agreed. I don't want to do this to my daughter. I chose my husband. I met him when I was eighteen years old. We married and I'm happy. That is what I want for my daughter. She can marry whom she wants when she is older. Now she is just a little girl.

Kenza worked primarily in the smaller towns surrounding Agadir. She visited households on a regular basis and relayed the information that she learned from the training sessions at the RHO to local men and women, but she spoke mainly to women who did not hold employment outside of the home. She explained that she knows some of these women sew clothing or make crafts to be sold at the larger markets in Agadir for additional income for their families. Kenza stated, "I like what I do. I like working with women. I like that I can do this and be a mother. I can bring my children with me." I responded that it seemed she was extremely happy to be a mother to her children. She agreed and said, "Yes. I love having my children around me. They are like my friends, with me all the time."

Kenza's comments contradict the assumption that children negatively shape Moroccan women's identities and how they think of themselves as citizens, as argued by feminist scholars mainly in the 1970s and 1980s, such as Vanessa Maher (1974) in *Women and Property in Morocco*. Maher calls the situation that Kenza described restrictive and asserts that it has negative influences over women's identity formation. Maher notes that many Moroccan women's children might range in age because women may have their firstborn children in their late teens or early twenties and they may continue to have children until they are in their late thirties. This implies that for a woman "there are always children around her, dependent on her for care and attention and greatly reducing her mobility. So it is that most of her activities must be carried out within a severely circumscribed space" (1974, 107). Whereas this claim certainly holds weight for certain segments of Morocco even today, Kenza did not buy into the conjecture that having children was a negative and severely restricting aspect of a woman's life. Although the birthrate in Morocco has dramatically decreased since the time Maher conducted her study, motherhood was far from a biological activity for Kenza.

In an attempt to understand how Kenza positions herself as a mother within the development agenda in Morocco, I asked about her children's futures and what she wanted for them. She started her response by mentioning that she wanted both of her children to pass the *baccalaureate* examination and to receive their high school diplomas.[2] Kenza sees herself playing an important role in the development of Morocco through raising her children. She stated, "I am important" when I inquired how she feels mothers participate in building the country's future. She said this very matter-of-factly, as if I had almost posed a challenge to her significance. She continued, "I will send my kids to school. I cook for them and I clean the house. I wash their clothes. All of this is important. This is all hard work. Who will do this for them?" She noted children are the future of Morocco, "That is why what I do every day at home and as a volunteer is very important. I can teach women things too. They wouldn't learn it from other places." Kenza took great pride in being a mother and raising the next generation of modern citizens and in teaching other mothers how to do the same.

By this time a second woman joined the conversation, Meryem. She was also a volunteer for the RHO. She was born in Morocco but spent time living in Saudi Arabia because of her husband's job. Meryem had three children and stated that she wanted to stay in Morocco rather than return to Saudi Arabia to raise them. She asked Kenza if she had children, then she turned to me to ask the same question. I responded that I did not have children at the time. She then asked, "Why not? How old are you?" I said that I was twenty-six, but I was not ready to become a mother just yet. I stated that I did want to have children in the future, inshallah. Meryem had a puzzled look on her face as if twenty-six seemed like a late age to begin having children. She explained, "You will become a woman when you have children. You will understand life. Children are the most important thing for us." Kenza and Meryem made motherhood seem as though it was simple, obvious, and transparent, even though it is in reality fraught with difficulties and contradictions. I discovered that all of the sixteen women who were in attendance that day for the training session were mothers, with the minimum number of children being two. Even the cleaning lady explained that she took the job to help support her children's education because even though she was never formally educated, she did not want her children to end up the same way.

Contradictions have played a central role in the scholarship on motherhood in the MENA (Eickelman 1992; Kanaaneh 2002). To a certain extent, Kenza and Meryem's comments echo Bourqia's (1995) findings that having children contributes to the ways that women define themselves and how their bodies and existence are constructed in Moroccan society. Kenza's comments point to a combination of national development discourses surrounding women's roles and the social configurations of women that exist in Morocco. The INDH places great emphasis on producing specific types of future citizens through women's childrearing practices, which begin in the hospital the moment they give birth. Whereas development stresses the importance of women's roles in the family and grants them greater responsibility in producing the future nation, Kenza has not internalized this rhetoric in a negative fashion as Maher suggests. Instead, she contradicts it and demonstrates that the Moroccan society Maher discussed may not even exist today. Kenza recognizes the extreme importance of her mothering practices in the creation of the nation-state. Phrases such as "I am important" and "Who will do that" allude to her awareness of her prescribed role as a woman within development and, at the same time, captures the importance of mothering as a form of production, not solely reproduction.

## LAYLA: A HOUSEWIFE AND PROVIDER

"You don't want five children like me," said Layla to her daughter Sarah one evening. This came after Sarah explained that she wanted a big family like her own, which included her, two sisters, and two brothers. When I asked why Sarah should not have several children like she wanted, Layla responded that in Morocco it is just too difficult to raise many children. "I am always busy cleaning and cooking," she stated. Layla lives in a one-bedroom apartment with her husband and children in a working and middle-class neighborhood in Rabat. She shares the only bedroom with her husband, and the children sleep in one of the two sitting rooms in the apartment. The family took in foreign students as a form of income even though the father works as a security guard with the government and is a former army official. However, his income is still not enough to support all of the children and his wife. When I inquired whether or not hosting students was a burden on Layla, she responded that she urged her husband to allow students to stay in their home in order to make money and to send their children to good schools in the future. Four of the children attended public school for their *baccalaureate*, and the oldest son, the second child, was sent to an international private school in Rabat because he spent his days hanging out with friends instead of being in class. After failing the *baccalaureate* exam twice, the public school refused to admit him for his final year due to his poor attendance record and his parents had to find another school for him.[3]

Two of the children were attending college at the time, and the middle daughter was about to start school to become a dental hygienist. Her dream was to attend university in France to study literature. Layla explained that when her daughter was ready to go and her papers were in order, she would be sure to have the money to pay for her tuition and to support her. Layla described herself as an equal financial contributor to the family by taking in students but as the main provider for her five children in terms of ensuring they had food and clothing in addition to a good education. One day Layla explained to my friend and me in private that she was very upset with her husband because he was not helping the children succeed in their education or find jobs. A week or so before, I had accompanied the family to drop off the oldest son so he could take the entrance exam for the military medical school. Being a military doctor was one of the most prestigious and well-paying government positions in the country. Layla was not confident in her son's abilities and wanted her husband to bribe *(soudoyer)* the officials so that their son could enter the program. Her husband had refused. She explained that one of the main reasons she takes in students is to pay such corruption money when needed and to help her daughter make it to France in order to attend college. Layla said her husband is not attentive when she tries to discuss their daughter's plans with him. He believed it was up to God and that God will make sure their children receive a proper education and find good jobs in the future. Whereas Layla considers herself to be a good Muslim, she was skeptical of this. Layla said to us as tears welled up in her eyes, "God will not pay the money. God will not pay for her stay in France. My husband won't. I have to do it." From further conversations with Layla, it was clear that she understood her children must meet high expectations in terms of education and training to find a well-paying job in Morocco, a country that she described as being plagued with economic problems and corruption.

In her own eyes, Layla is a nurturer and caregiver for her children, and she gives instructions about the proper ways to raise a family, such as those she provided to Sarah. At the same time, she is the one who will ensure her children's happiness and future through taking on added responsibility in order to save money for their education. Layla tests her own body and strength by taking in foreign students and having to provide additional meals for them as well as cleaning their rooms and doing their laundry. She often described herself as *'iyana* (tired) all the time because of these added duties, but in return, she was able to help financially support her children. (Although, having additional bodies in the apartment made it very difficult for the children to have a quiet place or any quiet time to study.) For Layla, being a responsible mother came at the price of her own health. On several occasions when I visited the family, she was ill. She suffered from colds frequently and would nap in the afternoons, which she said helped relieve the aches and pains. And although the three daughters would help cook and clean, especially during school holidays, Layla thought it was more important for them to study. She told the foreign students who stayed at their home, "You are here to study. I am a housewife. I will do the cooking and cleaning. You just study."

For Layla, fatigue serves as a marker of her level of responsibility of a mother. She identifies herself as being accountable to her children no matter what the trade-off may be, even if it means her health. Even though she declared to me many times that she was a good Muslim woman, she was unsure that God will truly be able to fulfill the needs of her children in terms of education and jobs. One afternoon I inquired as to what she understands a good Muslim woman to be. She explained that it is through specific Islamic practices, such as prayer, which she and her daughters did regularly in their home, and even more so through practices that are in her opinion Islamic, but may be questionable by others (Göle 1996), including wearing the hijab when traveling outside of the home and not allowing daughters to date or marry without the consent of the father and eldest brother. For her, being a good Muslim woman was much more through everyday practice than it was through a belief system, but her husband insisted that Islamic virtues be instilled in their children through religious education in school and within the home. In part, this included reading the Qur'an on a daily basis and teaching the children not to participate in corruption and to have faith in God's will.[4] However, Layla tested this when she was caught stealing money from the foreign students who stayed in the family's home. When confronted with this accusation by the organization that placed students with the family, her explanation was that the students did not pay her enough for all of the work she had to do even though they were from Europe and the United States. In addition, she explained that she was the one who needed to save money for her children's future.

Layla's story is complex. One the one hand, she sacrifices her own health in order to take care of her children. On the other hand, she defies the very Islamic principles that her husband insists they instill in their children. Layla's description of the wear on her body due to the extra work within the home attests to her high level of responsibility, but at the same time, she picks and chooses what is considered to be ethical and moral behavior. Not being able to fulfill her daughter's dreams of going to France or her son's plans of becoming a doctor is deemed as being irresponsible by Layla, but stealing money from students in order to make this happen seems to raise less concern.[5] This is not to say that Layla does not deal with contradictions in her own ways nor am I attempting to psychologize her, but, rather, I want to point out that she creates her own set of ethics that guide her choices of which childrearing practices to deploy and which to not. Layla proclaimed several times over the course of our relationship that she was a good Muslim woman, but she challenged the values her husband declared to be Islamic in order to satisfy her own Islamic principles, which included caring for her children and making their aspirations possible.

To analyze Kenza, Meryem, and Layla's stories, I in part draw on feminist standpoint theory, which proposes that women's experiences in society are fundamentally different from those of men and thus women's lives need to be a main point of departure. Feminist scholars suggest that women tend to understand the world in a manner that is different from men (Behar and Gordon 1995). What I attempt to do here is to discern what responsibility is in terms of childrearing for Moroccan women and how they identify themselves as being responsible mothers in the midst of various sources of information and instruction about mothering, some of which were described in the previous section. Giving birth has been described by feminist standpoint theorists as one of the "invariant and *nearly* unchangeable" (Ruddick 1980, 364; original italics) parts of life, whereas childrearing "is clearly a societal choice" (Hartsock 1983, 289). There is often a slippage here between essentialized women's experiences circumscribed by biological aspects and the plethora of social constructions of motherhood (Haraway 1989). Kenza, Meryem, and Layla all identify themselves as straddling the borderline between the biological and the social. Whereas the national policy circumscribes women's roles in development as mainly controlling the fertility rate and population growth, these three women have transformed such roles as they take on greater responsibility in raising future generations that are physically healthy, well educated, and able to secure employment within Morocco, albeit the practices by which they go about doing this may differ.

## THE DESIRED CHILD: ECONOMICALLY RESPONSIBLE AND "HAVING A GOOD HEART"

Over the course of my fieldwork, women expressed to me their various constructions of the desired child. Overall children should be healthy, well fed, educated, and intelligent. This is so that they can grow up to lead a successful professional as well as moral life as adults. El Shakry suggests within national discursive formations, the positioning of women is "an articulatory practice that [seeks] to construct women, by protecting, advancing, or developing them as *both* as a domain of culture . . . and progress" (1998, 130; original italics). The case of Morocco, I think, highlights El Shakry's observation. Women in Morocco have been identified by the state and development organizations as a "sphere of transformation." They are designated as such because they have the abilities to shape the future generations through their mothering. The inclusion of children into a national collective is far from a pure biological phenomenon, even though it may start there. Women and children often come to represent the collective's identity, which requires and creates a need to discipline the body along with the mind (Foucault 1995).

In my observations of women as well as in my conversations, I suggest that revisions to the development agenda in addition to major political regime changes in Morocco have become evident in mothering practices and are also illustrated by the particular children that women should and desire to raise. Data collected from interviews with women in both their early and later reproductive years illustrate this point because the characteristics that their children are to possess sometimes varied. Childrearing served as an important means through which my female participants expressed their visions of the future Morocco and articulated their ideas of what changes need to be made within the current political and social systems in order to suit the everyday needs of citizens.

As he took the throne, King Mohammed VI brought about a new set of development goals that focused on the enhancement of Moroccan citizens' lives. His new policies made women and youth central, which is evident from the Human Development Report (*50 Ans de Développement Humain et Perspectives 2025).* This shift from economic objectives to social development has certainly played a role in the ideology by which mothers are to mold their children's behaviors and minds. However, I argue that women's conceptions of the desired child have also changed as the state shifted its focus for development from economics to human development. In my research I found that younger women did not particularly discuss children purely in terms of economic investment for their own futures as much as older women did. I am not stating that this is not an important factor for them, but rather pointing out that their emphasis was more on the importance of raising a child who will be happy and successful and who will lead a good and moral life.[6] Younger women emphasized the need for children to have morals and to grow up to be responsible for their actions; these are attributes that are to be learned through being well versed in Islamic texts and principles, not just through the state's neoliberal development rhetoric.

Saouda, a twenty-three-year-old woman, and I met at the RHO's clinic in Zitounia. One day we were sitting in the waiting room with her two-year-old daughter, Aziza. The three of us sat together and Saouda and I chatted while she waited to see the OB/GYN for a consultation. She could not find someone to watch her daughter that morning while she was gone, so she brought Aziza with her, who actually occupied herself most of the time while sitting on Saouda's lap. Her husband worked in the neighborhood at a local community organization, and she was very cautious that we did not leave the clinic during our first few meetings because she was unsure if her husband would approve of her being seen with a foreign woman in public. I asked Saouda when Aziza would start school. She told me she would attend kindergarten when she is five years old. The school is actually very close to their home, which is not far from the clinic. I just nodded. Saouda went on to say that Aziza will begin preschool even sooner. I asked if the school is private or public, and she responded that it was a program run through one of the local mosques. I inquired about the class, asking about the students and the subject matter. Saouda said such programs are very popular in the area and Aziza was fortunate to have a place in the local program for it is normally full every year. At the mosque both young boys and girls will attend classes for just a few hours a week in order to learn simple verses from the Qur'an and Islamic principles. Aziza will receive basic religious instruction prior to beginning her education in the public Moroccan system.

On one occasion when I interviewed an Imam at a mosque in central Morocco, I actually walked into one of these classes for children by mistake as I was trying to find the library where our interview was to take place. Young children, boys and girls, sang songs based on the verse from the Qur'an they had learned that week from their teachers. As our interview continued you could hear them singing and reciting very short passages from the Qur'an. You could also hear the children laugh during the pauses. When I asked the Imam about what I was listening to, he just responded with a smile that "they are learning." Saouda stated such classes were very important for Aziza and for children in Morocco in general. I asked why exactly and she responded at public school she would be exposed to many different children and several new ideas, some of which may not be of the proper nature. She wanted Aziza to "have a good heart" (*q'lb mzyan*), and she would only gain this through attending the classes at the mosque. She said it is the heart that counts and what people believe; it is not so much about how they dress (she referred to wearing an abaya) or how intelligent they are. For Saouda, to succeed and to get ahead in life, Aziza must have this groundwork in Islam upon which she can build. I asked if Aziza would have Islamic studies in the public school, as all Moroccan children did for several years. Saouda responded that she would just like any other child, but she wanted to give her an even better foundation by enrolling her in these classes at a very young age. Aziza would learn everything else much quicker in her opinion if she learned verses from the Qur'an and other Islamic texts first, before heading to public school.

Having her daughter lead a moral life was extremely important for Saouda. This morality was based in Islam, and, more specifically, it was based upon Aziza's understanding of the sacred texts and Islamic values rather than practices, such as wearing the abaya in public, which may not be directly sanctioned by Islamic legal scholars in Morocco. These diverse practices are often termed as popular Islam in Morocco and in Muslim communities worldwide. Saouda expressed this foundation in Islam is necessary due in part to her lack of confidence in the public school system in Morocco, which has fallen under great criticism by the majority of the population as not preparing students properly for further education or the working world. I have heard firsthand stories from students whose teachers did not show up for class for an entire week or who would need to pay teachers for "extra hours" after school because they refused to teach the materials needed for exams during regular class time.[7] In addition, by being able to select the preschool program she sends her daughter to, Saouda is able to partially control the Islamic rhetoric that Aziza is being taught by individuals other than herself. Even though she recognizes that students receive Islamic instruction in public school, Aziza will be with a diverse group of students, which may influence the religious information that she receives or impact how she interprets such instruction while being exposed to children from different upbringings and statuses.

Besides being in good health, having a solid foundation in the Islamic texts and principles is one of the most important attributes that children can posses for Saouda. She as a mother feels it is her duty to provide this. By doing so, Aziza will then have "a good heart," which will enable her to live morally. Hajjer, the executive staff member at the RHO, is married to a man who works for the government and is fortunate enough to send her children to the private French school in Rabat. In one of our conversations, Hajjer began to discuss her youngest daughter having a boyfriend who lived in their neighborhood. I asked what she thought of this, and she said that she did not mind. Her daughter Anissa was responsible because she was brought up Muslim. In fact, Hajjer said that she was happy in part because the boyfriend's mom drove the children to school every morning and she did not have to worry about her daughter walking or taking the public bus. I asked Hajjer what exactly she meant when she stated her daughter was responsible. Was this because she and her husband raised her to be a good Muslim woman? She explained to me that within the home, she and her husband ensure that their daughters understand the behaviors that a Muslim woman should exhibit. This was not just any Muslim woman in her opinion; she described a "modern" (*moderne*) Muslim woman who could study in a private school and be taught by French and Canadian teachers but yet retain certain elements of her Moroccan heritage, most importantly Islam. Anissa will not follow Islamic classes in school, and therefore the instruction within the home and the example that her parents set are even more essential. According to Hajjer, this foundation in "modern" Islamic principles is necessary in order for Anissa to become a successful adult in the future, not just financially but also personally.

Hajjer has a slightly different definition of the desired child than Saouda. Whereas Saouda emphasized the importance of her daughter learning Islamic texts, Hajjer focused on practices that are considered to be proper for females. Some are considered to stem from the Qur'an, such as the importance of virginity and women not having sexual relations with men until they are married, whereas others may be questioned as to whether or not they are socially constructed behaviors in Morocco. For example, although Anissa may ride with her boyfriend and his mother to school, Hajjer would never allow Anissa to go over to his house nor would she allow him to visit her at their home as this would not be appropriate. They may visit the local PAUL, a very upscale café located near the French school, where foreigners tend to congregate for coffee or Sunday brunch, but never without a large group of male and female friends and never without Hajjer's or her husband's permission. Hajjer is seen as challenging the social barriers by allowing her daughter to have a boyfriend, which does not concern her or her husband because Anissa was taught Islamic values regarding how to behave as a woman. For Hajjer, morality includes knowing how to conduct oneself in a proper fashion, stemming from prescribed gender roles within Islam.

## LOOKING TOWARDS THE FUTURE

Children have long been theorized as important economic and social investments for women. This held true in several conversations I had with older Moroccan women. They expressed the need for their children to help support them in whatever way possible, even though it may not be much. For many of these women, the willingness to help their parents or their recognition of being indebted to their mother and father for raising them was a crucial attribute that children are to exhibit. Underlying older women's statements is the implication that children are an economic investment, an investment that offers returns when parents are unable to meet their own needs financially. This implication may in part be connected to the strict economic growth policies under which older women gave birth as their children were in their thirties and forties at the time of our conversation.

One female patient's mother who had seven grown children mentioned that her oldest daughter was a "good child" because she paid for her brother's education and would send gifts and money to the family from her home in Germany when she could. Jahira, the mother of Layla's husband, said to me on one of her visits to the family's home about her oldest son, "He has a family, but helps us, too. He was in the army. I know his sons will do the same for him and Layla." The patient's mother and Jahira emphasized that the "good child" would be able to care for their parents in their later years. It is for this reason that children should be well educated when they are younger. They should have the opportunity to develop skills that would help them in the workforce later on in life.

Morocco focused on economic growth until the 1990s, pushing for reforms that prioritized economics over social development. The overarching belief was that economic growth would lead to the improvement of social indicators, and this belief lasted until Morocco came under international scrutiny starting in the early 1990s as improvements to women's rights, education, poverty, and literacy were slim to none in comparison to other Arab countries. The family was (and continues to be) a key driver in economic development with remittances being sent back to Morocco from abroad, such as the case of the patient's sister, and children securing jobs in order to take care of their parents in times of need, like Jahira's son. This focus on financial gains certainly plays out in the stories of older women who gave birth and raised their children primarily under such strict economic policies.

Younger women like Saouda and Hajjer have taken on a slightly different outlook on the desired child. Their emphases were not so much on the economic returns that children can bring to the family, although this certainly may play a role, but rather on the morality of the child. Whereas they differ as to how this morality is learned or what it means, both Saouda and Hajjer expressed its importance as a characteristic that children should possess. These women have primarily raised their children under social development policies in Morocco where the stress is on fostering new mentalities in citizens and changing attitudes. For them, a major part of this new citizen is his or her ability to possess a set of morals and ethics that are based upon various aspects of Islam—the texts and the practices or popular Islam—which will culminate appropriate behaviors. Their methods of childrearing and their constructions of the desired child serve as political statements as they become expressions of women's envisioning of the future Morocco. Future generations, the foundation of the country, are to be given the tools and training in order to be successful financially but in a morally correct manner. Women articulated that this is in response to their frustration with the current political situation in Morocco, where they see corruption and dishonesty as running rampant and the status quo. They communicated that leaders will not follow through on promises, such as taking care of the poorer population or providing better education for children. For them, raising children to embody good morals is a way to counter their dissatisfaction and to change the country's future.

## CONCLUSION

Childrearing is far from an individual practice; it is intimately connected to public policies and political discussions on a national and international scale in Morocco and throughout the world (Mooney 2009). Rima Apple points out that parenthood today is "virtually synonymous with worry. We want to ensure that our children are healthy—physically, mentally, and emotionally" (2006, 1). Whereas Apple focuses primarily upon the science involved in childrearing in the United States, I found this worry to be prevalent among Moroccan women as they engaged in the medical system and in development in order to produce the future generations. This chapter has traced the sources from which women are educated, the ways that women speak of themselves as mothers, and the types of sons and daughters they hope to have. In doing so, I have demonstrated that the current development policy and the emphasis on the individualized self has not only produced new ways to mother and new definitions of motherhood that are debated in places like the waiting rooms, but it has also produced anxiety among working-class Moroccan women concerning how they are going to make this happen. Whereas women are finally recognized as being central to development, their new centrality is also a point of major ambivalence given it is due to their potential as mothers. The conclusion of this ethnography discusses this anxiety and focuses mainly on Moroccan children's bodies. It begins with a traumatic event, the closing of an orphanage because the government charged the foreign workers as attempting to convert the children to Christianity. Whereas I have focused primarily on women and mothers in the preceding chapters, the concluding chapter raises questions about how the state is constructing children within development and the future Morocco.

# Conclusion

## The Body, Uncertainty, and the Future of Morocco

The focus of this ethnography has been on how women's bodies and their childbearing and childrearing practices are used as vehicles by the Moroccan state, development agencies, and medical staff to create a modern nation and on the multitude of meanings women in Rabat have given to reproductive practices. In this conclusion, I would like to step outside of this framework for just a brief moment in order to use the events from the Already Loved Orphanage to question how children are being incorporated into the government's agenda for the creation of the modern citizen. After my discussion of the orphanage and the devastating events that occurred there, I will engage with broader discussions of reproductive technologies and modernization in the Muslim world and the need to analyze the processes surrounding them in nuanced ways. In addition, my concluding comments will illustrate how women feel an uncertainty when it comes to the future of their own bodies and their children because of the added social, political, and economic pressures put on them to raise modern and neoliberal future generations who will actively participate in Moroccan society. They are now expected to make responsible choices and to self-regulate their fertility in order to be "good" mothers and citizens, but sometimes this is difficult to do given their financial resources and social situations.

One day the Already Loved Orphanage in a small Moroccan village was raided by the military and government officials and was immediately shut down. The workers, most of them foreign born and Christian, were charged with trying to convert Muslim children to Christianity. Rather than dormitory style, the orphanage was set up so families would foster children. Each family had to make a ten-year commitment to live in Morocco to raise the orphans as their own. The families and workers I met while conducting research were from South Africa, the United States, New Zealand, and England, among other places. Some that had come and gone were also from other countries in Europe. Many of them had their own children who moved with them and acted as brothers and sisters to the children they fostered. All of the children attended a school run by the orphanage that was open to the public. The students received instruction in Arabic, English, and French from both Moroccan and international teachers. One worker,

Jonathon, explained to me that they tried to send the children to the public school in the nearby town, but their peers mocked them because they did not have mothers and fathers. Jonathon told me, "Teachers thought that the kids cannot learn above a third-grade level, so they didn't want to teach them anymore. The children cannot even get an education because they're orphans. That's why we opened up the school. We have local officials' children even attending." The Moroccan state signed the children over to the care of the orphanage as official adoption is illegal in Morocco due to Islamic sanctions concerning heritage, bloodlines, and opposite-sex siblings who technically could marry given they are not related through kinship.[1] Children can be fostered, as Islam expects you to help those who are less fortunate, but they cannot be officially adopted.[2] All of the families, teachers, and workers at Already Loved worked with the government in order to ensure all children were cared for properly and legally. The raid was a surprise to the workers, the children, the families, and to many people in the local area.

In her study of ophrans and secret adoption in Morocco, Jamila Bargach writes,

> It is, therefore, the womb that breeds backwardness, regardless of the fact that Morocco is a pro-natalist culture. Regress, in this case, is associated even with the abundance of those legally, religiously, and social sanctioned births, especially when those happen to be those births amongst the lower social strata, so one's imagination may never stray too far in imagining the kind of guilt, anathema, and marginalization associated with the uncontrollable womb that breeds even more backwardness in the form of unruly and unwanted bastards. (2002, 16)

Bargach points out that it is women's reproduction—their wombs—that not only produce future generations of modern citizens, but can also create those who are unwanted and do not fit within the ideal model of citizenship in Morocco. How are children's bodies being constructed by the state? How do their bodies problematize or exemplify the construct of the modern citizen put forth by the current development agenda? How is the future written on women's and children's bodies? There is a contradiction in the Moroccan state's plan. Through political acts, such as revising the Family Code and removing pictures of the veil from public school textbooks because it could be considered a marker of Islamic extremism, the government at the time of my fieldwork equated the liberalized state with a shift away from religion. But in this instance, the supposed threat of having future citizens become Christian was too much for the government to bear and it took action by closing down the orphanage. In the name of Islam and Moroccan law, the government reclaimed boys and girls who were unwanted and whose existence was not legally recognized due to the absence of their biological parents. I suggest that this is another strategic move that not only problematizes the construction of the citizen as hegemonic throughout Morocco, but it also further emphasizes the fact that Morocco is undergoing extremely rapid political and cultural transitions, all of which take place within the realms of kinship, the family, the body, and reproduction.

What was thought to be a routine check by the government authorities turned into a day that many people at Already Loved will never forget. Military accompanied the local officials, who explained to the workers and the parents they had just a few hours to pack up their things and to say good-bye to their children before they were deported. Over twenty people were deported the following day from Morocco only to be told to never enter the country again. When foreign parents first arrive, they all must sign a contract stating they will not break any of the country's laws, including proselytizing, while living there and engaging in the orphanage's work. Trying to convert someone from Islam to another religion is punishable by a fine and a jail sentence in Morocco, and in this case, being deported if you are a foreigner.[3] Since the events at Already Loved, Morocco has deported numerous Christians, such as missionaries and humanitarian workers. Whereas the constitution allows for religious freedom, individuals thought to be trying to convert Moroccans face serious consequences. There are several churches in the country (Catholic, Protestant, and non-denominational), and up until the mid-twentieth century, Morocco had a rather large Jewish population.[4] Videos of that day show the families at Already Loved crying as they said good-bye to their children.[5] Young boys and girls are hysterical in these clips because they do not understand why their parents, the only parents they have known, are being taken away from them. They cried and shouted. You can see some of the adults crying as well as they clung to the children. The orphanage often took in children with handicaps and debilitating illnesses, such as HIV/AIDS. Jonathon, my main contact at the orphanage, explained that he and his family were not deported, because they did not house any children themselves, but were required to move from the village where they were working with refugees the last time we spoke. He said that every day they wonder if they will be next on the list for deportation, even though they have lived in the country for several years. In written correspondence about the events, he asked me to keep in mind the children "whose existence is not recognized in their own society."

Why did the government reclaim the orphans at Already Loved if they were not legally recognized? If their very essence was not legitimate in the country, then why were they so important? A blogger from Rabat wrote on his page that social workers raised children who were rejected by their mothers, families, and the state for a variety of reasons (i.e., physical or mental disabilities, born out of wedlock, HIV positive). The blogger argues that even though these workers were Christian, it cannot be just assumed they were trying to convert the children from Islam. Another Moroccan blogger charges Already Loved happened because the government was trying to grab the attention of more conservative Muslims, who the blogger terms "Islamists." In expelling Christians who may have (or may not have) been trying to convert the children to Christianity, the Moroccan government was able to speak to the demands of Islamic groups in the country and also abroad. This event is certainly not isolated given the international controversy surrounding the supposed kidnapping of children from Haiti in the midst of the 2010 earthquake relief efforts. American missionaries were arrested for trying to take the children out of Haiti without the proper documentation. A news story stated that the missionaries in Haiti said they "did it in the name of Jesus Christ" (Moran 2010). Similarly, the event at the orphanage wraps Morocco up in international discussions of Islamic extremism, human trafficking, development, gender, and reproduction.[6]

The families of the children have made pleas with King Mohammed VI "to act with mercy" and to help the government and the organization reach a compromise so that the children at Already Loved can be reunited with the only parents they knew. So far, this has not worked as the parents have yet to be brought back together with their sons and daughters. A Moroccan court has ruled that there is sufficient evidence for a full trial and the case will go to court in the future to determine what will happen to the nearly thirty children from the orphanage. (All foreign workers were deported during the raid.) Already Loved is certainly a political move by the government in order to quell tensions that exist with Islamic groups and parties and to possibly situate Morocco as a strong ally with other Muslim majority countries in the MENA given its ambivalent positioning in the past.[7] Nevertheless, there are two interesting themes occurring here that are relevant to this ethnography. The first is that such political statements are being carried out not just upon Moroccan women's bodies, but also on the bodies of its future citizens. However, it is also women's bodies that bear future citizens who are unwanted and abandoned, left in the care of places like Already Loved. As noted by Bargach, women's reproductive bodies are critical to the production of these individuals—they must be managed and educated by the state and other agencies in order for productive and ideal modern citizens to be created. The second point is that Islam has become a marker of the future citizen. Even though these children were born to mothers out of wedlock or have been rejected by their biological families, the state is more concerned that they will no longer be Muslim by living with foreign parents.[8] The events at Already Loved begin the conclusion to this ethnography appropriately because they problematize the image of a liberalizing "moderate" Muslim nation-state that Morocco attempts to create for itself through policy revisions, reproductive choice, women's rights, and changes to the ideal family and to citizenship.

The introduction of reproductive technologies and healthcare has mixed effects on target populations. Inhorn and Sargent (2006) note that even though Islam is one of the fastest-growing religions in the world, in the West there is relatively little understanding of Islam and Muslim communities.

They write, "medical anthropology has much to contribute to discussions of Muslims' lives, as well as to greater understandings of Islam itself, a religion that can be said to encourage the use of medicine, biotechnology, and therapeutic negotiation and agency in the face of illness and adversity" (2006, 1). The female participants in my study discussed reproductive healthcare, and particularly the use of contraception, as having favorable and unfavorable consequences. As this ethnography has demonstrated, the Moroccan state has placed a great deal of responsibility on women for producing healthy and educated children who hold good morals and will grow up to become productive future citizens of the nation. Sensible reproductive practices and choices are critical to the modernization process; however, the working-class women I worked with did not have the same access to private doctors or schools for their children as some of the wealthier individuals. I noticed that a lack of financial resources combined with an overall absence of income-generating opportunities made it difficult for these women to raise such children. It also caused them to become more anxious about their children's futures because they were not able to give their children the material items or financial support that upper-class families could.

As I have shown in the previous chapters, women did not particularly view reproductive healthcare as a means to become autonomous self-sufficient citizens even though this rhetoric is found in popular and medical discourses. Rather, reproductive healthcare and family planning is a way for them to cope with the everyday trials of life as working-class individuals. This still falls in line with the neoliberal rhetoric of development in Morocco because my female participants placed the burden of national enhancement on themselves through the use of reproductive healthcare and not the state; continued to participate in modernization in a responsible manner; and believed that their choices will not only impact themselves, but their families and children. Models of women's citizenship in contemporary Morocco focus on planning, control, and accountability in terms of health, childbearing, and childrearing.

In nearly all of the family planning counseling sessions that I witnessed, Fatima stated that contraception can help women become less fatigued and can help their families economically. By spacing pregnancies or limiting their number of children, their bodies are able to rest and they can conserve their financial resources. I observed Fatima connect the state's rhetoric of modernization with women's reproductive healthcare by suggesting that using such services will improve their lives and their children's lives. She wanted women to learn that they must take care of themselves so they can take care of their families and ensure that they are well-fed, dressed properly, and developing intellectually and emotionally. Women must work hard to guarantee their children measure up to new standards set by the Moroccan government, which could produce wear and tear on their bodies and deplete their financial resources if they were of the working class. Contraception in particular can mitigate these issues by allowing women to recover after birth, to space their pregnancies, to take care of their children properly, and to invest larger amounts of money into a fewer number of children.

Fatima stated she also feels tired sometimes because of working to support her family and the physical labor involved in childrearing. This is why she used contraception to space her pregnancies and why she advocated for other women to use it as well. The RHO supported and encouraged women who work outside of the home and contribute to their household incomes, a large reason why it offered the sewing classes at the Tarma clinic. Whereas she and her husband hoped to have one more child, she wanted to wait for a period of time in order to let her body recover from childbirth and the wear on it from caring for her toddler, Ahmed. When I asked her how long she wanted to wait before having another child, she stated another year or two. Ahmed needed too much of her attention, and she could not handle caring for an infant and a toddler at the same time while also working full-time outside of the home. Having children too close in age could prohibit the older one from receiving the attention that he or she needs, thus slowing his or her physical and mental development.

During the counseling sessions, Fatima told women that they should wait a few years in between pregnancies, and to guarantee this, they must use contraception. In her advice, Fatima promotes similar messages as the Moroccan government—contraception and reproductive healthcare in general is a moral and necessary thing to do. She often emphasized to me and to medical staff that women, not the state and not other individuals, must bear the burden when it comes to childbearing and childrearing, which includes making sure that infants and children grow up to be healthy adults through proper nutrition, clothing, and education. Fatima stressed these are high expectations for the majority of women who came to the clinic as they do not have a vast amount of money. It is quite a burden for those women who have fewer resources at their disposal, which can in turn place greater strain on their own physical, mental, and emotional health.

The women who attended the clinics were concerned with the cost of raising children. It is very expensive in relation to their incomes, a point emphasized by Fatima during counseling. They would not be able to provide a large number of children with the tools they need to live up to the standards of success set for future generations by the development agenda in Morocco. In fact, this was not an uncommon response from women I met in the clinics. One woman in her midtwenties expressed fear her daughter would need to leave Morocco to find a job. She stated, "My husband's family lives in Italy. They moved there for work because there is not work here. My daughter may have to go, too, but I want to send her to a good school so she can find a job here in the future." By ensuring her daughter was well educated, this young mother believed she would have a better chance at finding a good-paying job in Morocco. From these women's stories, it is evident that contraception is a way for Moroccan women to offset financial burdens involved in producing the future citizens desired by the state. Contraception, particularly among those who do not have plentiful financial resources, is crucial to the production of such children as it allows them to carry out their national duty as citizens successfully.

Reproductive healthcare involves more than just medical practices for Moroccan women, as illustrated throughout this ethnography. Medical practices of reproduction take on multiple meanings within a society (Bourqia 1996), and sometimes this includes quelling anxieties that stem from women's perceptions of the educational system and professional opportunities in the country, configuring religious identities and new interpretations of Islam, and easing physical stress created by the need to enable the future generation of citizens that the Moroccan state hopes for. I do not dismiss the women who discussed the physical effects of reproductive healthcare with me, such as pain from the IUD or skin blotches from the birth control pill. As with any medical practice, adverse effects are certainly possible, but I also want to state that reproductive practices have great psychological and emotional purposes. Such practices become a way for women, although certainly not the only one, to speak out; to express their fears, concerns, excitement, and frustrations about the modern nation-state that Morocco is becoming; and to talk about issues they face in daily life surrounding childbearing and childrearing. Women demonstrated to me that reproductive healthcare is not only positive in their lives, but it can be an expression and source of their uncertainty as they are recognized as central actors in the modernization process and crucial to the global image that Morocco is building for itself.

In his article on the practice of infant bloodletting in Tajikistan, Salmaam Keshavjee writes, "As cultural products, both the construction and the experience of illness are subject to the vagaries and uncertainties of the social world and have contested meanings that exist within a web of cultural complexity informed by historical, religious, political, economic, and social experience" (2006, 72). He goes on to write about his approach to studying childhood illness: "I invoke a critical anthropology that presents local health conditions, institutions, and practices in terms of larger political and economic forces that shape and condition social life" (ibid.). Rather than examining infant bloodletting as purely a local folk practice, Keshavjee locates it within a complex matrix of social, religious, and cultural discourses and within the history of the post–Soviet Union. Keshavjee, along with other scholars who focus on the Middle East or on Islam (Clarke 2009; Inhorn 2006; Inhorn and Sargent 2006; Sargent and Cordell 2003), makes a call for more ethnographic research to be conducted on the nuances of medical practices in the region and how religious beliefs and practices intersect with medicine in mundane or profound ways. Johnson-Hanks states, "Much remains to be learned about the fertility of Muslims in specific times, places, and contexts" (2006a, 26). My hope is that this ethnography has helped to fill this theoretical and empirical void by offering insight into the childbearing and childrearing practices of urban Moroccan women and the national and global policies and rhetoric that shape them.

Similar to Keshavjee's approach, instead of locating reproductive practices at only the local level, I have found it much more productive in this project to understand them more broadly in terms of cultural forces, politics, religion, and economics. In particular, I have attempted to analyze how such practices fit within the agenda for modernization in Morocco, while at the same time I have tried to comprehend how the state's rhetoric of development is being filtered to working-class women in Rabat through the same practices.

As Hannah Arendt contends, "The distinction between a private and public sphere of life corresponds to the household and the political realms, which have existed as distinct, separate entities at least since the rise of the ancient city-state" (1958, 28). She continues, "the dividing line" between the private and the public is "blurred, because we see the body of peoples and political communities in the image of a family whose everyday affairs have to be taken care of by a gigantic, nation-wide administration of housekeeping" (ibid.). Women's wombs and their reproductive practices have long been at the center of the debate surrounding the role of the state in individuals' affairs and in civil society (Ginsburg 1998; Luker 1991), and often they have become the symbol of the nation for many (Kanaaneh 2002; Yuval-Davis 1997). I argue that on the one hand Moroccan women's wombs can be considered unruly and in need of regulation because they can produce children who are not wanted by society, such as those who were placed at the Already Loved Orphanage and then later taken back by the government. On the other hand, women's wombs can be viewed as critical to enhancing the nation and to producing children who will grow up to become exemplary modern citizens. It is through proper medical care and education about childbearing and childrearing, such as the information provided at the medical facilities where I conducted research, that women can produce and raise such citizens. The later view is documented in the development report *50 Ans de Développement Humain.* Since the launch of the INDH in 2005, women have been granted more responsibility for producing the modern nation. I am not suggesting that the state is completely absent from the frame nowadays, but rather I want to propose that responsibility for proper childbearing and childrearing has been reworked with a greater deal of it being placed on women's shoulders.

This book has sought to ethnographically investigate what this responsibility means for urban Moroccan women in their everyday lives and historically contextualize reproductive health and development in the country. Whereas the majority of the text has demonstrated that women give meanings to reproductive practices and appropriate them in ways that lie outside the intentions of the state, this conclusion has pointed to the uncertainty and anxieties concerning the future of Morocco and their children that added responsibility stirs up in them. With the coming of the INDH and neoliberal development reform, along with the desire to be a more prominent player in the world financial game, a need arose in Morocco to create a population that is active in their own governance, responsible, and self-regulatory—in other words, a population that is "modern" and can handle greater economic responsibilities. I have been primarily concerned in this book with the processes surrounding reproductive healthcare that work to create such citizens and have paid attention to the nuances of women's experiences. As Kamran Asdar Ali points out in the Middle East, "women's inclusion in the national community has also historically been determined differently from that of men, as women have remained hostages to particularistic discourses about cultural authenticity" (2002, 167). Women play a key role in the modernization agenda in Morocco, and the process of creating modern citizens begins at a place that is unruly and uncontrollable and yet at the same time is imperative and essential—the womb.

# Notes

## NOTES TO THE PROLOGUE

1. These are both pseudonyms, as are all the names used in this book for people and places. In addition, I have altered the names of some of the institutions I worked at during my fieldwork.
2. My friend also discussed "visa rings" that set up American or European citizens with Moroccans. A middleman would arrange for the Moroccan to pay a certain fee, and then he or she would find a foreign citizen for him or her to marry. The American or European would then be paid for the marriage. From our conversations, this tended to be between older foreign women and younger Moroccan men.

## NOTES TO THE INTRODUCTION

1. Deborah Caulfield Rybak, "Morocco," *Delta Sky Magazine*, March 2010, 69.
2. "Moroccan Islamists Sentenced to Death," *BBC News*, July 12, 2003, accessed September 8, 2012, http://news.bbc.co.uk/2/hi/africa/3060747.stm.
3. According to the Population Reference Bureau (2012), countries categorized as "more developed" have a natural rate of increase at 0.1 percent, those categorized as "less developed" are at 1.4 percent per year on average, and countries ranked as "least developed" have a natural rate of increase at 2.4 percent per year.
4. "Fertility Rate, Total Births per Woman," World Bank, accessed September 9, 2012, http://data.worldbank.org/.
5. The population of Rabat is 1,622,900 as of 2004, and the population of Casablanca is 3.5 million, making it the largest city in the country.
6. All conversion rates are as of March 2012. This rate of course fluctuates, but I want to give a general idea of how much it costs.
7. "Over USD 300 Million to Improve Living Conditions in Rabat Area," June 20, 2005, accessed September 8, 2012, http://friendsofmorocco.org/2005News/June05/0626News.htm#Over%20USD%20300%20million%20to%20improve%20living%20conditions%20in%20Rabat%20area.
8. This is a long loose robe often worn in Morocco when in public. It has long sleeves and a hood. Women would wear djellabas while walking on the streets or at the market and then remove them once they entered their home.

## NOTES TO CHAPTER 1

1. Karen Edwards, "Travel Eye: Fall in Love with Casablanca," *Huffington Post*, August 3, 2012, accessed August 31, 2012, http://www.huffingtonpost.co.uk/karen-edwards/casablanca-travel-eye-fall-in-love-w_b_1728192.html?utm_hp_ref=uk.
2. Dominique Lagarde, "La Fracture Morale," *L'Express*, May 6, 2008, 45–47.
3. For comparison, the maternal mortality rate for Egypt and Tunisia is sixty-six maternal deaths and fifty-six maternal deaths per one hundred thousand live births, respectively, as of 2012.
4. Morocco operates under a constitutional monarchy. There are regular elections of government officials with certain positions, such as the prime minister, appointed by the king.
5. *Le Figaro* (2001), quoted in Cohen and Jaidi (2006, 1).
6. Discours Royal a l'Occasion du 52ème Anniversaire de la Révolution du Roi et du People, Tetouan, August 20, 2005, quoted in Cohen and Jaidi (2006, 2).
7. Devon Pendleton, "King of Rock," *Forbes*, June 17, 2009, accessed December 14, 2009, http://www.forbes.com/2009/06/17/ king-morocco-phosphate-business-billionaires-royal-conflict.html.
8. Mrs. Jones (USAID Morocco) in discussion with the author, April 2009.
9. UNFPA identified Morocco as a priority country for reproductive health and family planning, but dropped it in 1982.
10. See www.ippf.org/en.
11. Julia Beamish and Lina Tazi Abderrazik "Adolescent and Youth Reproductive Health in Morocco: Status, Issues, Policies, and Programs," POLICY Project, January 2003, accessed August 31, 2012, http://hivaidsclearinghouse.unesco.org/search/resources/bie_morocco_ youth_reproductive_health_en.pdf
12. See Vermeren (2002) and Sater (2007) for more on Moroccan political history. See "Espionage: The Murder of Mehdi Ben Barka," *Time*, December 29, 1975, for more on Ben Barka. He was a self-exiled critic of the former king Hassan II who disappeared in France. It has been confirmed, although still with some suspicion, that he was killed by three officials from Morocco, including Interior Minister Mohammed Oufkir, who was killed in 1972 after attempting to assassinate King Hassan II. The leftist party he led then split into several different factions but has continued its opposition of the monarchy.
13. *Istiqlāl* in Arabic means independence or freedom.
14. The main office of the RHO is located in Rabat and is composed of eleven executive staff members who oversee all of the operations throughout the country. This includes the executive director and his assistant, who have worked for the association for a combined eighteen years; a small financial department; the director of programs, who was promoted from overseeing the clinics in another region; the coordinator for the health clinics in the Rabat region; the manager of supplies nationally; the youth director (at first this was an older gentleman who worked part-time for the Ministry of Health, but now it is a younger man who used to work for the Ministry of Youth); and an office manager. As compared to other development organizations in Morocco, the RHO is relatively small in size.
15. The fee for services for adolescents is subsidized by the RHO and other international donor agencies.
16. Dr. Smith (Al Akhawayn University) in conversation with the author, September 2008.
17. Although important, HIV/AIDS and abortion fall outside of the scope of my project and therefore will not be discussed here as in-depth as the other three areas.

18. A large proportion of the population in Morocco is of *Amazigh* (Berber) origin. Amazigh language has different regional dialects: *tarifit*, *tamazight*, and *tachelhit*. Tamazight language (a term used to sometimes describe Amazigh language as a whole) has been incorporated into the curriculum into several primary schools, mostly where a considerable number of students speak a dialect at home.
19. There are strong political and social connotations surrounding the term "Berber," and I prefer to use *Amazigh* in this text. In Agadir, youth and adults speak one of the dialects known as Tachelhit widely at home and in public. Many youth at this training session spoke Tachelhit, but because not all did, the lessons were mainly in Moroccan Arabic and some French.
20. There were two military coups against the king during his reign. See Oufkir and Fitoussi (2001).
21. King Mohammed VI, "Address to the High-Level Meeting of the General Assembly Commemorating the 60th Anniversary of the Creation of the United Nations Organization," address given to the United Nations, New York, September 14–16, 2005.
22. Although he has been deemed the "king of the poor," it is estimated that his palace's daily operating cost is approximately one million dollars (Pendleton 2009). King Mohammed VI holds a PhD in law from the Université de Nice Sophia-Antipolis and has been awarded an honorary degree from George Washington University for his promotion of democracy in Morocco.
23. King Mohammed VI and Princess Lalla Salma have two children: a son born in 2003 and a daughter born in 2007.
24. "Morocco Lowers Voting Age," *BBC News*, December 11, 2002, accessed January 26, 2007, http://news.bbc.co.uk/2/ hi/africa/2565373.stm.
25. "Morocco: Giving Women More Rights," *Muslim Women's Coalition*, accessed November 12, 2009, http://www.mwcoalition.org/id130.html.
26. King Mohammed VI, "Address to the High-Level Meeting of the General Assembly Commemorating the 60th Anniversary of the Creation of the United Nations Organization."
27. See http://hdr.undp.org/hd.
28. Aristotle in ancient Greece even stated, "Wealth is evidently not the good we are seeking, for it is merely useful for the sake of something else." (*Nichomachean Ethics*, 350 BC).
29. See http://hdr.undp.org/hd.
30. The World Bank, http://data.worldbank.org/.
31. U.S. Department of State, "Background Note," March 12, 2012.
32. The Amazigh languages are spoken predominantly in southern Morocco, but also in the north.
33. In Rabat there are French and American primary and secondary schools. In Casablanca, there is an American academy. These are just to name a few. There are currently four international baccalaureate high schools as well.
34. Samanta Jay, "Education Reforms in Morocco," *ezinearticles*, accessed August25,2012,http://ezinearticles.com/?Education-Reforms-in-Morocco&id=1014496.

## NOTES TO CHAPTER 2

1. Henna is a dye used to decorate women (and men's) hands and feet for special ceremonies, like weddings or the birth of a child.
2. For instance, in Marrakech on any given day in the large square *Jam' al-fna'*, several women will be waiting with their henna pens to paint the hands of tourists.

3. See Russell, Thompson, and Sobo. (2000) for a discussion of traditional and modern methods of contraception.
4. Hajar Dehhani, "Contraception: Choisissez celle qui vous convient!" *Famille Actuelle*, March 2008, 83–85.
5. Wassim Rhazi Senhaji, "Interview: Chaque femme peut trouver une méthode de contraception adaptée," *Famille Actuelle*, March 2008, 86.
6. Mohamed Yacoubi, "Interview: Il est essentiel que la femme puisse contrôler son corps," *Citadine*, October 2008, 85.
7. Melanie Frerichs-Cigli, "On fait le point sur les nouvelles contraceptions," *Citadine*, October 2008, 83–84.
8. "Illiteracy Rate in Morocco Drops to 38.5%," *Magharebia*, April 20, 2007, accessed November 27, 2012, http://magharebia.com/cocoon/awi/xhtml1/en_GB/features/awi/ newsbriefs/general/2007/04/20/newsbrief-04
9. Kris (PhD student conducting fieldwork in Morocco) in conversation with the author, June 2008.
10. This is a handcrafted robe that is worn to special ceremonies like weddings.
11. This family only had the two main Moroccan channels at this time. They did not have satellite television that broadcast channels from around the world.
12. Minal Shwaqī, "Nhaya al-`alqa al-ḥmema bīn al-um wa el-ṭfl," *Magella al-mara al-Arabea: Sītadīn*, January 2008, 112–113.
13. Latifa Abousaid, "Votre Enfant," *Femmes du Maroc*, October 2008, 176.
14. Nafissa El Bouanani, "Grossesse: Haro sur les idées reçues!" *Citadine*, January 2008, 81.

## NOTES TO CHAPTER 3

1. The RHO outreach program is run through the clinics. Amin will gather supplies from different clinics depending on which rural area he will be traveling to. Whereas it is not directly part of the health clinics, I feel that it is important to discuss in this chapter because the program also contributes to the creation of modern responsible citizens in its own ways. In addition, some women from the outreach program will attend the clinics when they are pregnant or for yearly well-woman exams.
2. No matter what service women desired, the counselor would see them in the order in which they arrived. However, when two doctors were present at the same time, this required two different lines. Sometimes the counselors would give women a second number in the counseling room, depending on whether they were there to see the OB/GYN or the other specialist. They would use this number to line up for the doctor then. Also, women who would see the dermatologist or generalist would have a different type of chart. It tended to be smaller in size than those of women seeing the OB/GYN.
3. In the United States, insurance companies and healthcare providers often offer parents similar books for infants. Blue Cross Blue Shield provided my parents with the *Health and Immunization Record* book when I was born. My mother recorded all of my immunizations and other important health information in this book, which I still have over thirty years later.
4. Mr. Benjalli explained that after women complete the literacy course for Arabic they can move onto a course in French, but not as many will do this.
5. I will discuss the sewing classes in further detail and provide insight as to the participants' perspectives of them later in Chapter 6.
6. In the original article, Zemni and Bogaert refer to the INDH as NIDH, the English acronym for the program.

## NOTES TO CHAPTER 4

1. I was in Morocco for preliminary research in the summer of 2005 when Muslim suicide bombers coordinated attacks on public transportation in London during rush hour. Fifty-two civilians were killed in addition to the bombers and about seven hundred civilians were injured. One day I was speaking to a Muslim woman who worked at the center where I was studying Moroccan Arabic about the attacks. Her response to me was: "The people who did this are not Muslim. They do not know Islam. Islam is not about violence." It is important to remember that Islam is not homogenous or monolithic. There are multiple interpretations, some of which Muslims themselves do not agree with.
2. Zlotnik was the chief of the Mortality and Migration Section of the Population Division from 1993 to 1999 and she was also the director of the Population Estimates and Projections Section from 1999 to 2003. She served as the assistant director from 2003 to 2005. Before joining the division, she worked for the Committee on Population and Demography of the United States National Research Council.
3. Abortion garnered a tremendous amount of media attention in Morocco over the course of my fieldwork. Articles on abortion that discussed various sides of the debate appeared in numerous women's and news magazines, including *Femmes du Maroc*, *Citadine*, *Le Journal*, and *Telquel.*
4. For more on *ijtihad*, see Ali-Karamali and Dunne (1994), Hallaq (1984), and Ramadan (2008).
5. Abdallah S. Daar and A. Khitamy, "Bioethics for Clinicians: 21. Islamic Bioethics," *Canadian Medical Association Journal* 9(2001): 60–63.
6. Carla Makhlouf Obermeyer, "Reproductive Choice in Islam: Gender and State in Iran and Tunisia," *Studies in Family Planning* 25(1994): 41–51.
7. A 2008 article that appeared in the news magazine *Telquel* stated, "The PJD wants to take the initiative of organizing a parliamentary debate about abortion." Cerise Maréchaud, "Je ne comprends pas le silence des féministes," *Telquel*, October 11, 2008, 30.
8. The students raised the point that the conservative party was concerned that making such pill available would encourage sexual intercourse outside of marriage, which along with adultery, is forbidden by Islam.
9. In 2012, a young man was arrested for eating in public on the streets of Rabat. He was ordered to pay a fine. Article 222 of the Moroccan penal code punishes those who break the fast in public without a valid excuse. "Moroccan Sentenced for Breaking Ramadan Fast" *Al-Akhbar*, August 28, 2012, accessed September 4, 2012, http://english.al-akhbar.com/node/ 11523.
10. See El Guindi (1999), Laborde (2008), and Shirazi (2003) for more on the hijab and Muslim dress.
11. However, certain ethnic groups in Morocco are known for their lighter skin or their light eyes. *Rabatis*, or people from the capital Rabat, are thought to be descendants of the Spanish and French and are commonly referred to by their blue eyes or their blond hair. It is somewhat of a status symbol if you are a *Rabati* or marry into a *Rabati* family.
12. There is a similar passage in the Bible, "But every woman who prays or prophesies with her head uncovered dishonors her head—it is the same as having her head shaved. For if a woman does not cover her head, she might as well have her hair cut off; but if it is a disgrace for a woman to have her hair cut off or her head shaved, then she should cover her head. A man ought not to cover his head, since he is the image and glory of God; but woman is the glory of man. For man did not come from woman, but woman from man; neither was man created for woman, but woman for man" (1 Corinthians 11:5–9).

13. Richard Hamilton, "Moroccan Airline Bans Prayer Time," *BBC News*, November 6, 2006, accessed September 4, 2012, http://news.bbc.co.uk/2/hi/africa/6120324.stm.
14. She used the term *fular*. This is from the French word *foulard* meaning "(head) scarf." It is a square piece of material, but Moroccans commonly use the term to describe the hijab.
15. He referenced the beginning of Muslim prayers, "*Bismillah al-rahman al-rahim*" (In the name of God, most Gracious, most Compassionate).
16. The Maliki School of jurisprudence has followers in North Africa, West Africa, and other parts of the Middle East. The school comes from Medina and is named after Anas bin Malik, who lived from 717 to 801. It relies on the Qur'an, Sunnah in addition to the customs and practices of the people of Medina at the time it was formed, and the general welfare of the community for its rulings.
17. An abaya is a very loose fitting robe. It tends to cover the whole body except the face.
18. A niqab is a veil worn to cover the hair and face except for the eyes. In general, it is not very popular in Morocco, but it is worn by some women.

## NOTES TO CHAPTER 5

1. This phrase is like inshallah. Many different people utter both in various situations regardless of whether or not they are practicing Muslims. It could be more of a cultural saying than an actual religious statement.
2. The RHO relied mainly upon public events, press coverage, and referrals from hospitals and public health clinics in addition to word of mouth to attract new patients and promote its services.
3. This test is very similar to a pregnancy test that can be bought at most large chain retailers, grocery stores, and pharmacies in the United States.
4. hCG stands for human chorionic gonadotropin. It is a hormone that is produced by the developing placenta after conception. If a woman is testing after her expected menstrual cycle start date, she can test at later points in the day because enough hCG will have been produced by that point to produce a positive pregnancy test no matter what urine she uses. If she is testing on or before her expected menstrual cycle start date, then she should test only in the early morning given the higher concentrations of hCG at that time of the day.
5. When I say "correct" in this instance I am referring to Fatima's interpretation. From her reading and formal and informal religious education, she believes this is the standard interpretation that all believers should follow. I am not suggesting that there is only one "correct" reading here.
6. Mrs. Fisher (Al Akhawayn University) in conversation with the author, September 2008.
7. The counselors at the health clinics were literate. They could read and write in both Arabic and French because of their schooling and medical training and Fatima spoke some English as well. Both Fatima and Kaoutar were well versed in Islam and often prayed and read the Qur'an during the afternoon lunch break.

## NOTES TO CHAPTER 6

1. Men did attend the RHO clinics to see the dermatologist or the family physician themselves. Men tended not to accompany women when they came to

see the OB/GYN or another specialist. Some of them did wait in the waiting room, but this was not only uncomfortable to them, but to the women as well. They could not breastfeed their babies in front of men who were unrelated, and they had to replace their niqabs if non-kin men were present.

2. See Lobna Flah, "Bac Math Exams Leaked on Facebook, 617 Cheating Cases across the Country," *Morocco World News*, June 13, 2012, accessed September 12, 2012, http://www. moroccoworldnews.com/2012/06/44116/bac-math-exam-leaked-on-facebook-617–cheating-cases-across-the-country-ministry/.
3. Students may take the exam three times but must repeat the entire school year before they are allowed to retake it.
4. Part of the PJD's platform is to work on corruption in the government. "The PJD's Islamist Government starts to 'Learn' How to Work with the King," *Rue 20*, accessed September 12, 2012, http://rue20.com/english/?p=538.
5. The head of the organization that placed students with the family wanted to press charges and get the police involved when she discovered what was happening. Stealing from the students placed in their home was not deemed an acceptable behavior.
6. See Cohen (2004) for more on global market integration and the affect such policies have on identity formation in Morocco.
7. For "extra hours" teachers would charge students extra fees for meetings after the school day. They would not teach what students are required to know for the exams during the day. The only way students could get this information was through attending these "extra hours," which would occur at a place other than schools.

## NOTES TO THE CONCLUSION

1. Marcia Inhorn, "'He Won't be My Son': Middle Eastern Muslim Men's Discourses of Adoption and Gamete Donation," *Medical Anthropology Quarterly* 20(2006): 94–120.
2. The verse from the Qur'an reads: "Allah has not made for a man two hearts in his interior. And He has not made your wives whom you declare unlawful your mothers. And he has not made your adopted sons your [true] sons. That is [merely] your saying by your mouths, but Allah says the truth, and He guides to the [right] way. Call them by [the names of] their fathers; it is more just in the sight of Allah. But if you do not know their fathers—then they are [still] your brothers in religion and those entrusted to you. And there is no blame upon you for that in which you have erred but [only for] what your hearts intended. And ever is Allah Forgiving and Merciful" (33:4–5).
3. According to the law, anyone who prevents another from attending worship services of any religion may be punished with a fine and a jail sentence. It is the same penalty for "anyone who employs enticements to shake the faith of a Muslim or to convert him to another religion." Anyone who is accused of this offense has a right to a court trial if he or she has lived in the country without incident for more than ten years. "July-December, 2010 International Religious Freedom Report," U.S. State Department, Bureau of Democracy, Human Rights, and Labor, accessed September 7, 2012, http://www.state.gov/j/drl/rls/irf/ 2010_5/168272.htm.
4. In 2005, Morocco even hosted a multiday Christian music festival featuring contemporary singers and bands (from the United States and abroad) in Marrakech.

5. I will not include the website links to these videos so not to disclose the exact location of the orphanage or the identities of the workers and children. I also will not include the direct citations of the blogs and websites that discuss the situation at the orphange for this reason.
6. To my knowledge, the Moroccan government did not make a statement linking the closing of Already Loved or the deporations of non-Muslims to the kidnapping charges in Haiti.
7. See Dan Wooding. "Moroccan Islamists 'Use Facebook to Target Christians,'" *Assist News Service*, June 17, 2010, accessed September 7, 2012, http://www.assistnews.net/Stories/ 2010/s10060099.htm. In the article, Wooding states the news agency learned that "Muslim extremists" were encouaging the government to seek out Moroccan Christians. Supposedly the group posted images of Christian converts and their families with derogitory terms attached to them and gave information as to their places of worship.
8. I want to note again that I conducted my fieldwork prior to the PJD winning the majority of seats in Parliament in late 2011. The events at the orphanage may have played out differently under this new government—either positively or negatively.

# Bibliography


Abu-Lughod, Lila. "Do Muslim Women Really Need Saving? Anthropological Reflections on Cultural Relativism and Its Others," *American Anthropologist* 104(2002): 783–790.

Adams, Alice. *Reproducing the Womb: Images of Childbirth in Science, Feminist Theory, and Literature.* Ithaca: Cornell University Press, 1994.

Agamben, Giorgio. *Homo Sacer: Sovereign Power and Bare Life.* Stanford: Stanford University Press, 1998.

Ahmed, Leila. *Women and Gender in Islam: Historical Roots of a Modern Debate.* New Haven: Yale University Press, 1992.

Al Arabiya and Agencies. "Morocco to Vote with Islamist Party Set for Strong Showing," *Al Arabiya News*, November 24, 2011. Accessed July 22, 2012, http://www.alarabiya.net/ articles/2011/11/24/179034.html.

Alarcón, Norma, Caren Kaplan, and Minoo Moallem. "Introduction: Between Woman and Nation." In *Between Woman and the Nation: Nationalisms, Transnational Feminisms, and the State*, edited by Caren Kaplan, Norma Alarcón, and Minoo Moallem, 1–18. Durham: Duke University Press, 1999.

Ali, Kamran Asdar. *Planning the Family in Egypt: New Bodies, New Selves.* Austin: University of Texas Press, 2002.

Ali-Karamali, Shaista and Fiona Dunne. "The Ijtihad Controversy," *Arab Law Quarterly* 3(1994): 238–257.

Althusser, Louis. "Ideology and Ideological State Apparatuses." In *Lenin and Philosophy and Other Essays*, translated by Ben Brewster, 121–176. Danvers: Monthly Review Press, 1971.

Andaya, Elise. "The Gift of Health," *Medical Anthropology Quarterly* 23(2009): 357–374.

Anderson, Benedict. *Imagined Communities: Reflections on the Origin and Spread of Nationalism.* New York: Verso Books, 1991.

Angrosino, Michael. "Catholic Social Policy and U.S. Health Care Reform: A Relationship Revisited," *Medical Anthropology Quarterly* 15(2001): 312–328.

Appadurai, Arjun. *Modernity at Large: Cultural Dimensions of Globalization.* Minneapolis: University of Minnesota Press, 1996.

Apple, Rima. *Perfect Motherhood: Science and Childrearing in America.* New Brunswick, NJ: Rutgers University Press, 2006.

Arendt, Hannah. *The Human Condition.* Chicago: Chicago University Press, 1958.

Ayad, Mohamed, and Farzaneh Roudi. "Fertility Decline and Reproductive Health in Morocco: New DHS Figures," May 2006. Accessed September 19, 2012, http://www.prb.org/Articles/2006/FertilityDeclineandReproductiveHealthin-MoroccoNewDHSFigures.aspx.

Bargach, Jamila. *Orphans of Islam: Family, Abandonment, and Secret Adoption in Morocco*. Lanham, MD: Rowman and Littlefield Publishers, 2002.

Barlow, Kathleen. "Critiquing the 'Good Enough' Mother: A Perspective Based on the Murik of Papua New Guinea," *Ethos* 32(2004): 514–537.

Barry, Andrew, Thomas Osborne, and Nikolas Rose, eds. *Foucault and Political Reason: Liberalism, Neo-Liberalism, and Rationalities of Government*. Chicago: University of Chicago Press, 1996.

Barthes, Roland. *Mythologies*. Translated by Annette Lavers. New York: Farrar, Straus and Giroux, 1972.

Bassin, Donna, Margaret Honey, and Meryle Mahrer Kaplan, eds. *Representations of Motherhood*. New Haven: Yale University Press, 1994.

Batnitzky, Adina. "Obesity and Household Roles: Gender and Social Class in Morocco," *Sociology of Health and Illness* 30(2008): 445–462.

Becker, Gay. "Metaphors in Disrupted Lives: Infertility and Cultural Constructions of Continuity," *Medical Anthropology Quarterly* 8(1994): 383–410.

Behar, Ruth, and Deborah A. Gordon, eds. *Women Writing Culture*. Berkeley: University of California Press, 1995.

Ben-Meir, Jason. "Royal Activities: King Seeks to Foster New Citizenship Mentality," *Morocco Times*, October 14, 2005. Accessed October 3, 2006, http:www.moroccotimes.com/paper/printArticle.asp?id=10278.

Berend, Zsuzsa. "Surrogate Losses: Understandings of Pregnancy Loss and Assisted Reproduction among Surrogate Mothers," *Medical Anthropology Quarterly* 24(2010): 240–262.

Bernal, Victoria. "Colonial Moral Economy and the Discipline of Development: The Gezira Scheme and 'Modern' Sudan," *Cultural Anthropology* 12(1997): 447–479.

Bledsoe, Caroline H., and Fatoumatta Banja. *Contingent Lives: Fertility, Time, and Aging in West Africa*. Chicago: University of Chicago Press, 2002.

Boddy, Janice. *Wombs and Alien Spirits: Women, Men, and the Zār Cult in Northern Sudan*. Madison: University of Wisconsin Press, 1989.

Body, Richard. "Religion and Discussion of End-of-Life Care: The Hunt for the Hidden Confounder Must Begin," *Journal of Medical Ethics* 37(2011):61.

Boellstorff, Tom. *Coming of Age in Second Life: An Anthropologist Explores the Virtually Human*. Princeton: Princeton University Press, 2008.

Bolognetti, Maurizio. É tempo di referendum. No all'ottusa e illiberale legge sulla procreazione assistita (Referendum Time: No to the Obtuse and Illiberal Assisted Reproduction Law). *Radicali Lucani* press release, March 13, 2004.

Bop, Coudou. "Islam and Women's Sexual Health and Rights in Senegal," *Muslim World Journal of Human Rights* 2(2005). Accessed February 14, 2011, doi: 10.2202/1554-4419.1032.

Bourqia, Rahma. "Women Uncertainty, and Reproduction in Morocco." In *Family, Gender, and Population in the Middle East: Policies in Context*, edited by Carla Makhlouf Obermeyer, 136–146. Cairo: American University of Cairo Press, 1995.

———. *Femmes et Fécondité*. Casablanca, Morocco: Afrique Orient, 1996.

Boutayeb, Abdesslam. "Social Inequalities and Health Inequity in Morocco," *International Journal for Equity in Health* 5(2006): 5–15.

Boutieri, Charis. "In Two Speeds (À Deux Vitesses): Linguistic Pluralism and Educational Anxiety in Contemporary Morocco," *International Journal for Middle East Studies* 44(2012): 443–464.

Bowen, Donna Lee. "Islamic Law and Family Planning." In *Islam and Social Policy*, edited by Stephen P. Hayneman, 118–155. Nashville: Vanderbilt University Press, 2004.

———. "Pragmatic Mortality: Islam and Family Planning in Morocco." In *Everyday Life in the Muslim Middle East*, edited by Donna Lee Bowen and Evelyn A. Early, 91–101. Bloomington: Indiana University Press, 1993.
Bray, Francesca. "Gender and Technology," *Annual Review of Anthropology* 36(2007): 37–53.
Brems, Eva. "Diversity in the Classroom: The Headscarf Controversy in European Schools," *Peace & Change* 31(2006): 117–131.
Bracke, Sarah. "Conjugating the Modern/ Religious, Conceptualizing Female Religious Agency: Contours of a 'Post-secular' Conjuncture," *Theory, Culture & Society* 25(2008): 51–67.
Brown, George F. "Morocco Family Planning Program: Progress and Problems," *Demography* 5(1968): 627–631.
Browner, Carole H. "Situating Women's Reproductive Activities," *American Anthropologist* 102(2001): 773–788.
Bruce, Steve. *Religion and Modernization.* Oxford: Oxford University Press, 1992.
Buckser, Andrew. *Communities of Faith: Sectarianism, Identity, and Social Change on a Danish Island.* Oxford: Berghahn Books, 1996.
Bullock, Katherine. *Rethinking Muslim Women and the Veil: Challenging Historical & Modern Stereotypes.* London: International Institute of Islamic Thought, 2002.
Burchell, Graham. "Liberal Government and Techniques of the Self." In *Foucault and Political Reason: Liberalism, Neo-Liberalism, and Rationalities of Government*, edited by Andrew Barry, Thomas Osborne, and Nikolas Rose, 19–36. Chicago: University of Chicago Press, 1996.
Burke III, Edmund. "Theorizing the Histories of Colonialism and Nationalism in the Arab Maghrib." In *Colonialism and Nationalism in the Maghrib,* edited by Ali Abdullatif Ahmida, 17–34. New York: Palgrave, 2000.
Burton, Laurel Arthur, and Marcia Sue Dewolf Bosek. "When Religion May Be an Ethical Issue," *Journal of Religion and Health* 39(2000): 97–106.
Calabrese, John. "Population Challenges and Economic Growth: Conference Summary," Middle East Institute, 2001. Accessed September 19, 2012, http://web.macam.ac.il/~arnon/Int-ME/ Population/ME%20Population.htm.
Cameron, Mary. "Feminization and Marginalization? Women Ayurvedic Doctors and Modernizing Health Care in Nepal," *Medical Anthropology Quarterly* 24(2010): 42–63.
Casper, Monica. "Reframing and Grounding Non-Human Agency," *American Behavioral Scientist* 3(1994): 839–856.
Chandrasekaran, C. and Albert I. Hermalin, eds. *Measuring the Effect of Family Planning Programs on Fertility.* Dolhain: Ordina Editions, 1975.
Chatterjee, Nilanjana, and Nancy E. Riley. "Planning an Indian Modernity: The Gendered Politics of Fertility Control," *Signs* 26(2001): 811–845.
Chesler, Phyllis. "Op-Ed: Let's Admit It: Honor Killing in the West is by Muslims," *Israel National News,* February 3, 2012. Accessed August 22, 2012, http://www.israelnationalnews. com/Articles/Article.aspx/11220#.UKvTHaVgPFI.
Clarke, Mari. "Pursing International Development through a Gender Lens," *National Association for the Practice of Anthropology Bulletin* 26(2006): 32–54.
Clarke, Morgan. *Islam and New Kinship: Reproductive Technology and the Shariah in Lebanon.* Oxford: Berghahn Books, 2009.
Cohen, Lawrence. "Where It Hurts: Indian Material for an Ethics of Organ Transplantation," *Daedalus* 128(1999): 135–166.
Cohen, Shana. *Searching for a Different Future: The Rise of a Global Middle Class in Morocco.* Durham: Duke University Press, 2004.

Cohen, Shana, and Larabi Jaidi. *Morocco: Globalization and Its Consequences.* New York: Routledge, 2006.

Cohen, Susan and Cory L. Richards. "The Cairo Consensus: Population, Development, and Women," *Family Planning Perspectives* 26(1994): 272–277.

Colen, Shellee. "'Like a Mother to Them': Stratified Reproduction and West Indian Childcare Workers and Employers in New York." In *Conceiving the New World Order: The Global Politics of Reproduction*, edited by Faye D. Ginsburg and Rayna Rapp, 78–102. Berkeley: University of California Press, 1995.

Collier, Stephen J., and Aihwa Ong. "Global Assemblages, Anthropological Problems." In *Global Assemblages: Technology, Politics, and Ethics as Anthropological Problems*, edited by Aihwa Ong and Stephen J. Collier, 1–21. Oxford: Blackwell Publishing, 2005.

Comaroff, Jean, and John Comaroff, eds. *Millennial Capitalism and the Culture of Neoliberalism.* Durham: Duke University Press, 2001.

Cooper, Richard S., Jay S. Kaufman, and Ryk Ward. "Race and Genomics," *New England Journal of Medicine* 348(2003): 1166–1170.

Courbage, Youssef. "Fertility Transition in the Mashriq and the Maghrib: Education, Emigration, and the Diffusion of Ideas." In *Family, Gender, and Population in the Middle East: Policies in Context*, edited by Carla Makhlouf Obermeyer, 80–104. Cairo: American University of Cairo Press, 1995.

Craven, Christa. "Claiming Respectable American Motherhood: Homebirth Mothers, Medical Officials, and the State," *Medical Anthropology Quarterly* 19(2005): 194–215.

Daaleman, Timothy P., and Larry VandeCreek. "Placing Religion and Spirituality in End-of-Life Care," *Journal of the American Medical Association* 284(2000): 2514–2517.

Davis, Dana-Ain. "The Politics of Reproduction: The Troubling Case of Nadya Suleman and Assisted Reproductive Technology," *Transforming Anthropology* 17(2009): 105–116.

Davis-Floyd, Robbie, and Carolyn F. Sargent. "Introduction: The Anthropology of Birth." In *Childbirth and Authoritative Knowledge: Cross-Cultural Perspectives*, edited by Robbie Davis-Floyd and Carolyn F. Sargent, 1–52. Berkeley: University of California Press, 1997.

Deeb, Lara. *An Enchanted Modern: Gender and Public Piety in Shi'i Lebanon.* Princeton: Princeton University Press, 2006.

———. "Emulating and/or Embodying the Ideal: The Gendering of Temporal Frameworks and Islamic Role Models in Shi'I Lebanon," *American Ethnologist* 36(2009): 242–257.

Degni, Filio, Charles Mazengo, Tuula Vaskilampi, and Britta Essén. "Religious Beliefs Prevailing among Somali Men Living in Finland Regarding the Use of the Condom by Men and that of Other Forms of Contraception by Women," *European Journal of Contraception and Reproductive Health Care* 13(2008): 298–303.

Diyen, Hayat. "Reform of Secondary Education in Morocco: Challenges and Prospect," *Prospects* 34(2004): 211–222.

Dwyer, Daisy. *Images and Self-Images: Male and Female in Morocco.* New York: Columbia University Press, 1978.

Eagleton, Terry. *Ideology: An Introduction.* London: Verso, 1991.

Ehrlich, Paul. *The Population Bomb.* New York: Ballantine Books, 1968.

Eickelman, Dale. *Knowledge and Power in Morocco: The Education of a Twentieth- Century Notable.* Princeton: Princeton University Press, 1992.

———. *The Middle East and Central Asia: An Anthropological Approach.* Upper Saddle River, NJ: Prentice Hall, 2002.

El Guindi, Fadwa. *Veil: Modesty, Privacy, and Resistance.* Oxford: Berg, 1999.

El Shakry, Omnia. "Schooled Mothers and Structured Play: Child Rearing in Turn-of-the-Century Egypt." In *Remaking Women: Feminism and Modernity in the Middle East*, edited by Lila Abu-Lughod, 126–170. Princeton: Princeton University Press, 1998.

———. *The Great Social Laboratory: Subjects of Knowledge in Colonial and Postcolonial Egypt*t. Stanford: Stanford University Press, 2007.

Ellison, James. "Governmentality and the Family: Neoliberal Choices and Emergent Kin Relations in Southern Ethiopia," *American Anthropologist* 111(2009): 81–92.

Elyachar, Julia. *Markets of Dispossession: NGOs, Economic Development, and the State in Cairo*. Durham: Duke University Press, 2005.

Engle-Merry, Sally. *Human Rights and Gender Violence: Translating International Law into Local Justice*. Chicago: University of Chicago Press, 2006.

Ennaji, Moha. "Language Contact, Arabization Policy and Education in Morocco." In *Language Contact and Language Conflict in Arabic: Variations on a Sociolinguistic Theme*, edited by Aleya Rouchdy, 70–89. New York: RoutledgeCurzon, 2002.

Erlanger, Steven, and Souad Mekhennet. "Islamic Radicalism Slows Moroccan Reforms," *New York Times,* August 26, 2009. Accessed July 23, 2012, http://www.nytimes.com/2009/08/27/ world/africa/27morocco.html?pagewanted=all.

Esposito, John. *What Everyone Needs to Know about Islam: Answers to Frequently Asked Questions from One of America's Leading Experts*. Oxford: Oxford University Press, 2002.

Farmer, Paul. "An Anthropology of Structural Violence," *Current Anthropology* 45(2004): 305–325.

Farquhar, Judith, and Qicheng Zhang. "Biopolitical Beijing: Pleasure, Sovereignty, and Self-Cultivation in China's Capital," *Cultural Anthropology* 20(2005): 303–327.

Ferguson, James. *The Anti-Politics Machine: "Development," Depoliticization and Bureaucratic Power in Lesotho*. Cambridge: Cambridge University Press, 1990.

———. *Global Shadows: Africa in the Neoliberal World Order.* Durham: Duke University Press, 2006.

Fernando, Mayanthi L. "Reconfiguring Freedom: Muslim Piety and the Limits of Secular Law and Public Discourse in France," *American Ethnologist* 37(2010): 19–35.

Fleuriet, K. Jill. "La Tecnologia y Las Monjitas: Constellations of Authoritative Knowledge at a Religious Birthing Center in South Texas," *Medical Anthropology Quarterly* 23(2009): 212–234.

Fordyce, Lauren. "Responsible Choices: Situating Pregnancy Intention among Haitians in South Florida," *Medical Anthropology Quarterly* 26(2012): 116–135.

Foucault, Michel. *The History of Sexuality: An Introduction*. New York: Vintage Books, 1990.

———. "Governmentality." In *The Foucault Effect: Studies in Governmentality,* edited by Graham Burchell, Colin Gordon, and Peter Miller, 87–104. Chicago: Chicago University Press, 1991.

———. *The Birth of the Clinic: An Archaeology of Medical Perception*. New York: Vintage Books, 1994.

———. *Discipline and Punish: The Birth of the Prison*. New York: Vintage Books, 1995.

Franzmann, Majella. "'God Desires Ease for You, and Desires Not Hardship for You': A Comparison of Qur'anic and Judaeo-Christian Law," *Islam and Christian-Muslim Relations* 21(2010): 1–9.

Galbraith, Marysia. "Choosing and Planning in a Climate of Insecurity: Balancing Professional Work and Family Life in Poland," *Journal of the Society for the Anthropology of Europe* 8(2008): 16–30.

Garcia, Angela. "The Elegiac Addict: History, Chronicity, and the Melancholic Subject," *Cultural Anthropology* 23(2008): 718–746.

Garrity, J.F. "Jesus, Peyote, and the Holy People: Alcohol Abuse and the Ethos of Power in Navajo Healing," *Medical Anthropology Quarterly* 14(2000): 521–542.

Gaylin, Willard. "Worshipping Autonomy," Hastings Center Report 26(1996): 43–45.

Gellner, Ernest. *Nations and Nationalism*. Oxford: Blackwell Publishing, 1983.

Georges, Eugenia. "Fetal Ultrasound Imaging and the Production of Authoritative Knowledge in Greece," *Medical Anthropology Quarterly* 10(1996): 157–175.

Gilligan, Carol. *In a Different Voice: Psychological Theory and Women's Development*. Cambridge: Harvard University Press, 1982.

Ginsburg, Faye D. *Contested Lives: The Abortion Debate in an American Community*. Berkeley: University of California Press, 1998.

Ginsburg, Faye D., and Rayna Rapp. "Introduction: Conceiving the New World Order." In *Conceiving the New World Order: The Global Politics of Reproduction*, edited by Faye D. Ginsburg and Raya Rapp, 1–17. Berkeley: University of California Press, 1995.

Goldstone, Jack. "The New Population Bomb: The Four Megatrends That Will Change the World," *Foreign Affairs* 89(2010): 31–43.

Göle, Nilufer. *The Forbidden Modern: Civilization and Veiling*. Ann Arbor: University of Michigan Press, 1996.

Gordon, Colin. "Governmental Rationality: An Introduction." In *The Foucault Effect: Studies in Governmentality*, edited by Graham Burchell, Colin Gordon, and Peter Miller, 1–51. Chicago: University of Chicago Press, 1991.

Gramsci, Antonio. *The Gramsci Reader: Selected Writings 1916–1956*. Edited by David Forgacs. New York: New York University Press, 2000.

Gravlee, Clarence C. "How Race Becomes Biology: Embodiment of Social Inequality," *American Journal of Physical Anthropology* 139(2009): 47–57.

Greene, Richard Allen. "Nearly 1 in 4 People Worldwide Is Muslim, Report Says," *CNN*, October 7, 2009. Accessed February 9, 2012, http://edition.cnn.com/2009/WORLD/ asiapcf/10/07/muslim.world.population/.

Greenhalgh, Susan. "Controlling Births and Bodies in Village China," *American Ethnologist* 21(1994): 3–30.

———. "Planned Births, Unplanned Persons: 'Population' in the Making of Chinese Modernity," *American Ethnologist* 30(2003): 196–215.

———. *Just One Child: Science and Policy in Deng's China*. Berkeley: University of California Press, 2008.

———. "The Chinese Biopolitical: Facing the Twenty-First Century," *New Genetics and Society* 28(2009): 205–222.

Greenhalgh, Susan, and Edwin Winckler. *Governing China's Population: From Leninist to Neoliberal Biopolitics*. Stanford: Stanford University Press, 2005.

Gremillion, Helen. *Feeding Anorexia: Gender and Power at a Treatment Center*. Durham: Duke University Press, 2003.

Grosse, Scott D. "The Politics of Family Planning in the Maghrib," *Studies in Comparative International Development* 17(1982): 22–48.

Hadley, Janet. *Abortion: Between Freedom and Necessity*. Philadelphia: University of Pennsylvania Press, 1996.

Hamilton, Richard. "Morocco Moves to Drop Headscarf," *BBC*, October 6, 2006. Accessed August 29, 2012, http://news.bbc.co.uk/2/hi/5413808.stm.

———. "Islamist PJD Party Wins Morocco Poll," *BBC*, November 27, 2011. Accessed September 20, 2012, http://www.bbc.co.uk/news/world-africa-15902703.

Hallaq, Wael B. "Was the Gate of Ijtihad Closed?" *International Journal of Middle East Studies* 16(1984):3–41.

Haraway, Donna. "Situated Knowledges: The Science Question in Feminism as a Site of Discourse on the Privilege of Partial Perspective," *Feminist Studies* 14(1988): 575–599.

———. *Primate Visions: Gender, Race, and Nature in the World of Modern Science.* New York: Routledge, 1989.

Harding, Sandra, ed. *Feminism and Methodology: Social Science Issues.* Bloomington: Indiana University Press, 1987.

———. "Rethinking Standpoint Epistemology: What Is 'Strong Objectivity'?" In *Feminist Perspectives on Social Research,* edited by Sharlene Nagy Hesse-Biber, 39–63. Oxford: Oxford University Press, 2004.

Haring, Kristen. "The 'Freer Men' of Ham Radio: How a Technical Hobby Provided Social and Spatial Distance, *Technology and Culture* 44(2003): 734–761.

Hartsock, Nancy. "The Feminist Standpoint: Developing the Ground for a Specifically Feminist Historical Materialism." In *Discovering Reality: Feminist Perspectives on Epistemology, Metaphysics, Methodology, and Philosophy of Science,* edited by Sandra Harding and Merrill B. Hintikka, 283–310. Dordecht: Kluwer Academic Publishers, 1983.

Harvey, David. *A Brief History of Neoliberalism.* Oxford: Oxford University Press, 2007.

Henderson, James W. *Health Economics and Policy.* Mason, OH: South-Western, 2009.

Hirschkind, Charles. *The Ethical Soundscape: Cassette Sermons and Islamic Counterpublics.* New York: Columbia University Press, 2006.

Hodgson, Dorothy L. *Once Intrepid Warriors: Gender, Ethnicity, and the Cultural Politics of Maasai Development.* Bloomington: Indiana University Press, 2001.

Hughes, Cortney. "The 'Amazing' Fertility Decline: Islam, Economics, and Reproductive Decision-Making among Working-Class Moroccan Women," *Medical Anthropology Quarterly* 25(2011): 417–435.

Huntington, Samuel. *The Clash of Civilizations and the Remaking of World Order.* New York: Touchstone, 1996.

Ibrahim, Azeem. "Muslims in America 2012—Who Will They Vote For?" *Huffington Post,* February 1, 2012. Accessed February 8, 2012, http://www.huffingtonpost.com/azeem-ibrahim/muslim-voters-2012_b_1247616.html.

Inhorn, Marcia. *Quest for Conception: Gender, Infertility, and Egyptian Medical Traditions.* Philadelphia: University of Philadelphia Press, 1994.

———. "Middle Eastern Masculinities in the Age of New Reproductive Technologies: Male Infertility and Stigma in Egypt and Lebanon," *Medical Anthropology Quarterly* 18(2004): 162–182.

———. "Religion and Reproductive Technologies: IVF and Gamete Donation in the Muslim World," *Anthropology News* 46(2005): 14,18.

———. "Medical Anthropology at the Intersections: Celebrating Fifty Years of Interdisciplinarity," *Medical Anthropology Quarterly* 24(2010): 263–269

Inhorn, Marcia, and Carolyn Sargent. "Medical Anthropology in the Muslim World: Ethnographic Reflections on Reproductive and Child Health," *Medical Anthropology Quarterly* 20(2006): 1–11.

Jabbra, Joseph G., and Nancy W. Jabbra. *Women and Development in the Middle East and North Africa.* Leiden: Brill Academic Publishers, 1992.

Jay, Martin. "New Prime Minister Surprises Moroccans With Support for Abortion," *New York Times,* January 11, 2012. Accessed September 13, 2012, http://www.nytimes.com/2012/01/12/world/africa/new-prime-minister-surprises-moroccans-with-support-for-abortion. html?pagewanted=all.

Jayawardena, Kumari. *Feminism and Nationalism in the Third World.* London: Zed Books, 1986.

Johnson-Hanks, Jennifer. "On the Politics and Practice of Muslim Fertility: Comparative Evidence from West Africa," *Medical Anthropology Quarterly* 20(2006a): 12–30.

———. *Uncertain Honor: Modern Motherhood in an African Crisis*. Chicago: University of Chicago Press, 2006b.

Jones, James W. "Religion, Health, and the Psychology of Religion: How the Research on Religion and Health Helps Us Understand Religion," *Journal of Religion and Health* 43(2004):317–328.

Jordan, Brigitte. "Authoritative Knowledge and its Construction." In *Childbirth and Authoritative Knowledge: Cross-Cultural Perspectives*, edited by Robbie Davis-Floyd and Carolyn F. Sargent, 56–80. Berkeley: University of California Press, 1997.

Joseph, Suad. *Intimate Selving in Arab Families: Gender, Self and Identity*. Syracuse: Syracuse University Press, 1999.

Kahn, Susan. *Reproducing Jews: A Cultural Account of Assisted Conception in Israel*. Durham: Duke University Press, 2000.

Kanaaneh, Rhoda. *Birthing the Nation: Strategies of Palestinian Women in Israel*. Berkeley: California University Press, 2002.

Kanna, Ahmed. "Flexible Citizenship in Dubai: Neoliberal Subjectivity in the Emerging 'City-Corporation,'" *Cultural Anthropology* 25(2010): 100–129.

Keefe, Susi Krehbiel. "'Women Do What They Want': Islam and Permanent Contraception in Northern Tanzania," *Social Science & Medicine* 63(2006): 418–429.

Keshavjee, Salmann. "Bleeding Babies in Badakshan: Symbolism, Materialism, and the Political Economy of Traditional Medicine in Post-Soviet Tajikistan," *Medical Anthropology Quarterly* 20(2006): 72–93.

Khosrowshahi, Cameron. "Privatizing in Morocco: The Politics of Development," *Middle East Journal* 51(1997): 242–255.

Kirsch, Thomas. "Restaging the Will to Believe: Religious Pluralism, Anti-Syncretism, and the Problem of Belief," *American Anthropologist* 106(2004): 699–709.

Kligman, Gail. *The Politics of Duplicity: Controlling Reproduction in Ceausescu's Romania*. Berkeley: University of California Press, 1998.

Konner, Melvin. *Medicine at the Crossroads: The Crisis in Health Care*. New York: Vintage, 1993.

Krause, Elizabeth. *Crisis of Births: Population Politics and Family-Making in Italy*. Belmont, CA: Wadsworth, 2005.

Krause, Elizabeth L., and Milena Marchesi. "Fertility Politics as 'Social Viagra': Reproducing Boundaries, Social Cohesion and Modernity in Italy," *American Anthropologist* 109(2007): 350–362.

Krieger, Nancy. "Embodiment: A Conceptual Glossary for Epidemiology," *Journal of Epidemiology & Community Health* 59(2005): 350–355.

Kridli, Suha Al-Oballi, and Kay Libbus. "Establishing Reliability and Validity of an Instrument Measuring Jordanian Muslim Women's Contraceptive Beliefs," *Health Care for Women International* 23(2002): 870–881.

Kum-kum, Bhavani."Tracing Contours: Feminist Research and Feminist Objectivity." In *Feminist Perspectives on Social Research*, edited by Sharlene Nagy Hesse-Bibler, 65–77. Oxford: Oxford University Press, 2004.

Laborde, Cecile. "Virginite et Burqa: Des Accommodements Deraisonnables? Autor des Rapports Stasi et Bouchard-Taylor," *La Vie Des Idees*, September 16, 2008. Accessed July 15, 2012, http://www.laviedesidees.fr/IMG/pdf/20080916_laborde.pdf.

Lakoff, Andrew. *Pharmaceutical Reason: Knowledge and Value in Global Psychiatry*. Cambridge: Cambridge University Press, 2005.

Langford, Jean M. "Gifts Intercepted: Biopolitics and Spirit Debt," *Cultural Anthropology* 24(2009): 681–711.
Layne, Linda. *Motherhood Lost: A Feminist Account of Pregnancy Loss in America.* New York: Routledge, 2003.
Lazreg, Marnia. *The Eloquence of Silence: Algerian Women in Question.* New York: Routledge, 1994.
Libbus, Kay, and Suha Kridli. "Contraceptive Decision Making in a Sample of Jordanian Muslim Women: Delineating Salient Beliefs," *Health Care for Women International* 18(2002): 85–94.
Liddell, James. "Morocco: Modern Politics or the Politics of Modernity?" Sada: Carnegie Endowment for International Peace, December 3, 2008. Accessed July 23, 2012. http://www.carnegieendowment.org/sada/2008/12/02/morocco-modern-politics-or-politics-of-modernity/6bje.
Liu, Lydia. *Translingual Practice: Literature, National Culture, and Translated Modernity China, 1900–1937.* Stanford: Stanford University Press, 1995
Lock, Margaret M., and Patricia Alice Kaufert, eds. *Pragmatic Women and Body Politics.* Cambridge: Cambridge University Press, 1998.
Lock, Margaret, Allan Young, and Alberto Cambrosio. *Living and Working with the New Medical Technologies: Intersections of Inquiry.* Cambridge: Cambridge University Press, 2000.
Lugo, Alejandro, and Bill Maurer, eds. *Gender Matters: Remembering Michelle Z. Rosaldo.* Ann Arbor: University of Michigan Press, 2000.
Luker, Kristin. *Taking Chances: Abortion and the Decision Not to Contracept.* Berkeley: University of California Press, 1991.
Mabilia, Mara. *Breast Feeding and Sexuality: Behaviour, Beliefs and Taboos among the Gogo Mothers in Tanzania.* New York: Berghahn Books, 2005.
Macfarquhar, Neil. "U.N. Sees Falling Middle East Fertility Rates." *New York Times*, April 3, 2009. Accessed February 27, 2011, http://dotearth.blogs.nytimes.com/2009/04/03/un-sees-big-drop-in-middle-east-fertility-rates/.
Macphee, Marybeth. "The Weight of the Past in the Experience of Health: Time, Embodiment, and Cultural Change in Morocco," *Ethos* 32(2004): 374–396.
Maddy-Weitzman, Bruce. "Population Growth and Family Planning in Morocco," *Asian and African Studies* 26(1992): 63–79.
Maher, Vanessa. *Women and Property in Morocco.* Cambridge: Cambridge University Press, 1974.
Marks, Loren. "Religion and Bio-Psycho-Social Health: A Review and Conceptual Model," *Journal of Religion and Health* 44(2006): 173–186.
Martín, I. "Morocco: The Bases for a New Development Model? The National Initiative for Human Development (INDH)," 2006. Accessed September 30, 2011, http://www. realinstitutoel cano.org/wps/wcm/connect/7869d7804f0186 e4bb8fff3170baead1/947_ Martin_MoroccoI.pdf?MOD=AJPERES&CACHEID=7869d7804f0186e4bb8fff3170baead1.
Maurer, William. *Mutual Life, Limited: Islamic Banking, Alternative Currencies, Lateral Reason.* Princeton: Princeton University Press, 2005.
Markens, Susan. *Surrogate Motherhood and the Politics of Reproduction.* Berkeley: University of California Press, 2007.
Marx, Karl. *Critique of Hegel's 'Philosophy of Right'*, edited by Joseph O'Malley, translated by Annette Jolin. Cambridge: Cambridge University Press, 1970.
McNay, Lois. *Foucault and Feminism: Power, Gender, and the Self.* Cambridge: Polity Press, 1992.
Mernissi, Fatima. "Obstacles to Family Planning Practice in Urban Morocco," *Studies in Family Planning* 6(1975): 418–425.
———. *Doing Daily Battle: Interviews with Moroccan Women.* New Brunswick: Rutgers University Press, 1988.

Mitchell, Timothy. *Rule of Experts: Egypt, Techno-Politics, Modernity.* Berkeley: University of California Press, 2002.

Mohanty, Chandra Talpade. *Feminism without Borders: Decolonizing Theory, Practicing Solidarity.* Durham: Duke University Press, 2003.

Montoya, Michael. "Bioethnic Conscription: Genes, Race, and Mexicana/o Ethnicity in Diabetes Research," *Cultural Anthropology* 22(2007): 94–128.

Mooney, Jagwiga E. Pieper. *The Politics of Motherhood: Maternity and Women's Rights in Twentieth-Century Chile.* Pittsburgh: Pittsburgh University Press, 2009.

Moran, Terry. "Kidnapping or Caring? Missionaries in Haiti Tried to Take Children to U.S. after Earthquake," *ABC News*, February 3, 2010. Accessed September 7, 2012, http:// abcnews.go.com/WN/haiti-earthquake-american-missionaries-arrested-kidnapping-children-proper/story?id=9736257#.UEokqk L3Bok.

Morell, Carolyn M. *Unwomanly Conduct: The Challenges of International Childlessness.* New York: Routledge, 1994.

Nelkin, Dorothy. "Science Controversies: The Dynamics of Public Disputes in the United States." In *Handbook of Science and Technology Studies,* edited by Sheila Jasanoff, Gerald E. Markle, James C. Petersen, and Trevor Pinch, 444–456. Thousand Oaks, CA: Sage Publications, 1995.

Newcomb, Rachel. *Women of Fes: Ambiguities of Urban Life in Morocco.* Philadelphia: University of Pennsylvania Press, 2008.

Nguyen, Vinh Kim, and Karine Peschard. "Anthropology, Inequality, and Disease: A Review," *Annual Review of Anthropology* 32(2003): 447–474.

Nussbaum, Martha. *Women and Human Development: The Capabilities Approach.* Cambridge: Cambridge University Press, 2001.

Obermeyer, Carla Makhlouf. "Reproductive Rights in the West and in the Middle East: A Cross-Cultural Perspective." I*n Family, Gender, and Population in the Middle East: Policies in Context*, edited by Carla Makhlouf Obermeyer, 1–15. Cairo: The American University of Cairo Press, 1995.

Olson, Emelie. "Muslim Identity and Secularism in Contemporary Turkey: 'The Headscarf Dispute,'" *Anthropological Quarterly* 58(1985): 161–171.

Omran, Abdel Rahim. *Family Planning in the Legacy of Islam.* London: Routledge, 1992.

Ong, Aihwa. *Neoliberalism as Exception: Mutations in Citizenship and Soverignty.* Durham: Duke University Press, 2006.

Ortner, Sherry. "Is Male to Female as Nature Is to Culture?" In W*oman, Culture, and Society*, edited by Michelle Rosaldo and Louise Lamphere, 67–87. Stanford: Stanford University Press, 1974.

Oufkir, Malika and Michèle Fitoussi. *Stolen Lives: Twenty Years in a Desert Jail.* New York: Miramax Books, 2001.

Parpart, Jane, Shirin Rai, and Kathleen Staudt, eds. *Rethinking Empowerment in a Global World: Gendered Perspectives.* London: Routledge, 2000.

Paxson, Heather. *Making Modern Mothers: Ethics and Family Planning in Urban Greece.* Berkeley: University of California Press, 2004.

Pence, Brian Wells, Philomena Nyarko, James F. Phillips, and Cornelius Debpuur. "The Effect of Community Nurses and Health Volunteers on Child Mortality: The Navrongo Community Health and Family Planning Project," *Scandinavian Journal of Public Health* 35(2007): 599–608.

Pendleton, Devon. "King of Rock," *Forbes,* June 17, 2009. Accessed July 12, 2011, http:// www.forbes.com/2009/06/17/king-morocco-phosphate-business-billionaires-royal-conflict.html.

Pennell, C. R. *Morocco since 1839: A History.* New York: New York University Press, 2000.

Peterson, Kristin. "Benefit Sharing for All?: Bioprospecting NGOs, Intellectual Property Rights, New Governmentalities," *PoLAR* 24(2001): 78–91.

Petryna, Adriana. "Ethical Variability: Drug Development and Globalizing Clinical Trials," *American Ethnologist* 32(2005): 183–197.

Pew Research Center. *Mapping the Global Muslim Population.* Washington, DC: Pew Forum on Religion and Public Life, 2009.

Phillips, James F, Wendy L. Greene, and Elizabeth F. Jackson. *Lessons from Community-Based Distribution of Family Planning in Africa.* New York: Population Council, Policy Research Working Paper, 1999.

Population Division of the United Nations. n.d. *Morocco: Abortion Policy.* Accessed September 4, 2012, http://www.un.org/esa/population/publications/abortion/doc/morocco.doc.

PRB. *World Population Data Sheet.* Washington, DC: Population Reference Bureau, 2012.

Rabinow, Paul. *French Modern: Norms and Forms of the Social Environment.* Chicago: University of Chicago Press, 1995.

———. *Reflections of Fieldwork in Morocco.* Berkeley: University of California Press, 1977.

Ramadan, Tariq. *Radical Reform: Islamic Ethics and Liberation.* Oxford: Oxford University Press, 2008.

Rapp, Rayna. *Testing Women, Testing the Fetus: The Social Impact of Amniocentesis in America.* New York: Routledge, 2000.

———. "Gender, Body, Biomedicine: How Some Feminist Concerns Dragged Reproduction to the Center of Social Theory," *Medical Anthropology Quarterly* 15(2001):466–477.

Rayner, Philip, Peter Wall, and Stephen Kruger. *Media Studies: The Essential Introduction.* London: Routledge, 2001.

———. *Media Studies: The Essential Resource.* London: Routledge, 2004.

Reed, Adam. "'My Blog is Me': Texts and Persons in UK Online Journal Culture (and Anthropology)," *Ethnos* 70(2005): 220–242.

Rich, Adrienne. "Compulsory Heterosexuality and Lesbian Existence," *Signs* 5(1980): 631–660.

Richey, Lisa Ann. *Population Politics and Development.* New York: Palgrave, 2008.

Rofel, Lisa. *Desiring China: Experiments in Neoliberalism, Sexuality, and Public Culture.* Durham: Duke University Press, 2007.

Rosaldo, Michelle Zimbalist. "Women, Culture, and Society: A Theoretical Overview." In *Woman, Culture, and Society*, edited by Michelle Zimbalist Rosaldo and Louise Lamphere, 17–42. Stanford: Stanford University Press, 1974.

Rose, Nikolas. *Powers of Freedom: Reframing Political Thought.* Cambridge: Cambridge University Press, 1999.

———. "Community, Citizenship, and The Third Way," *American Behavioral Scientist* 43(2000): 1395–1411.

Rose, Nikolas, and Peter Miller. *Governing the Present: Administering Economic, Social and Personal Life.* Cambridge: Polity Press, 2008.

Royaume du Maroc. *50 Ans de Développement Humain et Perspectives 2025.* Rabat: Royaume du Maroc, 2006.

Ruddick, Sara. "Maternal Thinking," *Feminist Studies* 6(1980): 342–367.

———. *Maternal Thinking: Toward a Politics of Peace.* Boston: Beacon Press, 1989.

Rudnyckyj, Daromir. "Spiritual Economies: Islam and Neoliberalism in Contemporary Indonesia," *Cultural Anthropology* 24(2009): 104–141.

Russell, Andrew and Mary Thompson. "Introduction: Contraception across Cultures." In *Contraception across Cultures: Technologies, Choices, Constraints,* edited by Andrew Russell, Mary Thompson, and Elisa J. Sobo, 3–26. Oxford: Berg, 2000.

Russell, Andrew, Mary Thompson, and Elisa Sobo, eds. *Contraception across Cultures: Technologies, Choices, Constraints,* Oxford: Berg, 2000.

Sadiqi, Fatima. "Morocco's Veiled Feminists," *Project Syndicate*, May 25, 2006. Accessed February 2, 2012, http://www.project-syndicate.org/commentary/morocco-s-veiled-feminists.

Said, Edward. *Orientalism.* New York: Vintage Books, 1979.

Sandelowski, Margarete. *With Child in Mind: Studies of the Personal Encounter with Infertility.* Philadelphia: University of Pennsylvania Press, 1993.

Sargent, Carolyn. "Reproductive Strategies and Islamic Discourse: Malian Migrants Negotiate Everyday Life in Paris, France," *Medical Anthropology Quarterly* 20(2006): 31–49.

Sargent, Carolyn, and Dennis Cordell. "Polygamy, Disrupted Reproduction, and the State: Malian Migrants in Paris, France," *Social Science & Medicine* 56(2003): 1961–1972.

Sater, James. *Civil Society and Political Change in Morocco.* New York: Routledge, 2007.

Sawyer, Suzanna. *Crude Chronicles: Indigenous Politics, Multinational Oil, and Neoliberalism in Ecuador.* Durham: Duke University Press, 2004.

Schaefer-Davis, Susan. *Patience and Power: Women's Lives in a Moroccan Village.* Cambridge: Schenkman Publishing Company, 1983.

Schaft, Gretchen. "Teaching Human Rights: Creating an Informed Citizenry in the Classroom," *Anthropology News* 51(2010): 27.

Scheper-Hughes, Nancy, and Margaret Lock. "The Mindful Body: A Prolegomenon to Future Work in Medical Anthropology," *Medical Anthropology Quarterly* 1(1987): 6–41.

Sen, Amartya. *Development as Freedom.* New York: Anchor Books, 1999.

Senturia, Kirsten. "A Woman's Work Is Never Done; Women's Work and Pregnancy Outcome in Albania," *Medical Anthropology Quarterly* 11(1997): 375–395.

Sharma, Aradhana. "Crossbreeding Institutions, Breeding Struggle: Women's Empowerment, Neoliberal Governmentality, and State (Re)Formation in India," *Cultural Anthropology* 21(2006): 60–95.

Shirazi, Faegheh. *The Veil Unveiled in Modern Culture.* Gainesville: University of Florida Press, 2003.

Sholkamy, Hania. "Procreation in Islam: A Reading from Egypt of People and Texts." In *Conceiving Persons: Ethnographies of Procreation, Fertility, and Growth*, edited by Peter Loizos and Patrick Heady, 139–159. London: London School of Economics Monographs on Social Anthropology, 1999.

Silverstein, Paul. "States of Fragmentation in North Africa," *Middle East Report* 237(2005): 26–33.

Sinding, Steven W., and Med Bouzidi. "Partnerships and Resources: Towards Cairo + 10; Achievements, Unfinished Business and New Challenges." In *Fifth Asian and Pacific Population Conference: Selected Papers*, UN Economic and Social Commission for Asia and the Pacific, 323–342. New York: UN, 2002.

Skalli, Loubna. *Through a Local Prism: Gender, Globalization, and Identity in Moroccan Women's Magazines*. Lanham, MD: Lexington Books, 2006.

———. "Women and Poverty in Morocco: The Many Faces of Social Exclusion," *Feminist Review* 69(2001): 73–89.

Slyomovics, Susan. "A Truth Commission for Morocco," *Middle East Report* 218(2001): 18–21.

Smith, Anthony D. *Nations and Nationalism in a Global Era.* Cambridge: Polity Press, 1995.

Smith, Sheila, and Desmond Cohen. "Gender, Development and the HIV Epidemic. HIV and Development Programme," UNDP, October 2000. Accessed October 16, 2011, http://www. usi.edu/business/cashel/346/DEVELOPMENT,%20 GENDER%20AND%20THE%20HIV%20EPIDEMIC.htm.

Speed, Shannon. "Dangerous Discourses: Human Rights and Multiculturalism in Neoliberal Mexico," *PoLAR* 28(2005): 29–51.

Spivak, Gayatri Chakravorty. "Can the Subaltern Speak?" In *Marxism and the Interpretation of Culture*, edited by Cary Nelson and Lawrence Grossberg, 271–313. Urbana: University of Illinois Press, 1988.

Stephenson, Rob. "District-Level Religious Composition and Adoption of Sterilization in India," *Journal of Health, Population and Nutrition* 24(2006): 100–106.

Sullivan, Deborah A. *Cosmetic Surgery: The Cutting Edge of Commercial Medicine in America*. New Brunswick, NJ: Rutgers University Press, 2001.

Sunder-Rajan, Kaushik. *Biocapital: The Constitution of Postgenomic Life*. Durham: Duke University Press, 2006.

Tawil, Sobhi. "Qur'anic Education and Social Change in Northern Morocco: Perspectives from Chefchaouen," *Comparative Education Review* 50(2006): 496–517.

Taylor, Janelle. "Big Ideas: Feminist Ethnographies of Reproduction," *American Ethnologist* 31(2004): 123–130.

Teman, Elly. *Birthing a Mother: The Surrogate Body and the Pregnant Self*. Berkeley: University of California Press, 2010.

UN. "Report of the International Conference on Population and Development," UN Population Division, Department of Economic and Social Affairs and the UNFPA, October 18, 1994. Accessed August 31, 2012, http://www.un.org/popin/icpd/conference/offeng/poa.html.

UNDP. *Human Development Report 2011. Sustainability and Equity: A Better Future for All*. New York: Palgrave Macmillan, 2011.

Unnithan, Maya and Kavita Srivastava. "Gender Politics, Development, and Women's Agency in Rajasthan." In *Discourses of Development: Anthropological Perspectives,* edited by R.D. Grillo and R.L. Stirrat, 157–182. Oxford: Berg Publishers.

Venema, Bernhard, and Jogien Bakker. "A Permissive Zone for Prostitution in the Middle Atlas of Morocco," *Ethnology* 43(2004): 51–64.

Vermeren, Pierre. *Le Maroc en Transition*. Paris: La Découverte, 2002.

Volk, Lucia. "'Kull Wahad la Hallu': Feelings of Isolation and Distress among Yemeni Immigrant Women in San Francisco's Tenderloin," *Medical Anthropology Quarterly* 23(2009): 397–416.

Wadud, Amina. *Qur'an and Woman: Rereading the Sacred Text from a Woman's Perspective*. Oxford: Oxford University Press, 1999.

Wall, Glenda. "Moral Constructions of Motherhood in Breastfeeding Discourse," *Gender & Society* 15(2001): 592–610.

Walmsley, Emily. "Raised by Another Mother: Informal Fostering and Kinship Ambiguities in Northwest Ecuador," *Journal of Latin American and Caribbean Anthropology* 13(2008): 168–195.

Waugh, Earle H. *Memory, Music, and Religion: Morocco's Mystical Chanters*. Columbia: University of South Carolina Press, 2005.

Weingartner, Laura. "Family Law Reform in Morocco: The Mudawana: Modernist Islam and Women's Rights in the Code of Personal Status," *University of Detroit Mercy Law Review* 82(2005): 687–713.

WHO. *Trends in Maternal Mortality: 1990 to 2010*. Geneva: WHO Document Production Services, 2012.

Winnicott, Donald. *The Maturational Processes and the Facilitating Environment.* London: Hogarth Press, 1965.
Winter, Bronwyn. *Hijab & The Republic: Uncovering the French Headscarf Debate.* Syracuse: Syracuse University Press, 2008.
Wozniak, Danielle. *They're All My Children: Foster Mothering in America.* New York: New York University Press, 2002.
Yuval-Davis, Nira. *Gender and Nation.* London: Sage Publications, 1997.
———. "Nationalism, Feminism, and Gender Relations." In *Understanding Nationalism*, edited by Montserrat Guibernau and John Hutchinson, 120–141. Cambridge: Polity Press, 2001.
Zemni, Sami, and Koenraad Bogaert. "Trade, Security and Neoliberal Politics: Whither Arab Reform? Evidence from the Moroccan Case," *Journal of North African Studies* 14(2009): 91–107.
Zhan, Mei. "Civet Cats, Fried Grasshoppers, and David Beckham's Pajamas: Unruly Bodies after SARS," *American Anthropologist* 10(2005): 31–42.
———. *Other-Worldly: Making Chinese Medicine through Transnational Frames.* Durham: Duke University Press, 2009.

# Index